The Biss Tribe:

Where You Activate Your Goddess Pleasure

Book 2 in The Biss Tribe Series

Elizabeth Ann Atkins

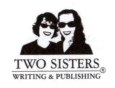

TWO SISTERS
WRITING & PUBLISHING

Copyrighted Material
The Biss Tribe: Where You Activate Your GoddessPleasure
By Elizabeth Ann Atkins
Copyright © 2024 Elizabeth Ann Atkins. All Rights Reserved.

No part of this publication may be reproduced, stored in a retrieval system or transmitted, in any form or by any means—electronic, mechanical, photocopy, recording, or otherwise—without prior written permission from the publisher, except for the inclusion of brief quotations in a review.

Disclaimer: If you have a serious mental or physical medical condition, please continue with your doctor's prescribed medical regimen and seek clearance before beginning the practices herein that include and are not limited to meditation, exercise and dietary changes.

The women attending the retreat are fictional characters.
Any similarity to actual people, living or dead, is purely coincidental.

For information about this title or to order other books and/or electronic media, contact the publisher:

Two Sisters Writing and Publishing
18530 Mack Avenue, Suite 166
Grosse Pointe Farms, MI 48236
www.TwoSistersWriting.com

ISBN-13: 978-1-956879-68-1 (Hardcover)
ISBN: 978-1-956879-69-8 (Paperback)
ISBN: 978-1-956879-70-4 (eBook)

Printed in the United States of America

Cover and Interior design: Van-garde Imagery, Inc.

Back cover author photo: Clarence Tabb, Jr. In My Eye Photography

Artwork and graphics created by Two Sisters Writing & Publishing®
on Adobe Firefly and Canva.

Pleasure is the Portal to your Power.

Dear Goddess Reader:

Before you read this book,
please read Book 1 in The Biss Tribe Series:

*The Biss Tribe: Where You Activate
Your GoddessPower.*

Available at TwoSistersWriting.com
and anywhere you buy books online.

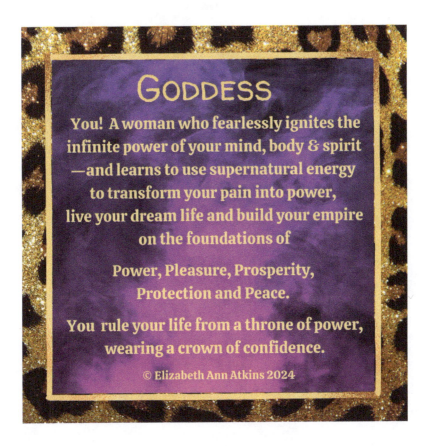

Welcome to The Bliss Tribe: Where You Activate Your Goddess Pleasure

Women's sexuality is the ultimate taboo.

It has been shamed, stifled and shut down throughout history.

Why? Perhaps because women have the power to create human life in our bodies. We are endowed with this miracle-making ability, and for that we have been feared and oppressed by the global patriarchy since the beginning of time, as it has sought to control our minds and bodies, and steal our Pleasure.

This emotional and physical domination has been so stealth, intricately woven into religion, family values and traditions, and societal standards, that it has locked the female psyche in a pleasureless prison of guilt, shame and fear where too many women remain sexually repressed for a lifetime.

Too many never orgasm. Or they don't engage in the many emotional and physical benefits of self-Pleasure. Or they don't liberate themselves to demand Pleasure in every way.

Now is the time for women everywhere to claim our divine birthright to enjoy and celebrate Pleasure as never before. This means seeking and savoring the sensuous thrills of our six senses: what we see, what we taste, what we touch, what we smell, what we hear, and what we feel with our intuition. This means pampering our minds and bodies with sensations and experiences that have scientifically-proven health benefits.

Welcome to The Biss Tribe

Yet too many women view themselves through the male gaze, always speaking, behaving, living and loving in a way that conforms to the rules imposed by religion, culture, families and society at large.

Breaking those rules can ruin a woman's reputation and career, and even cost her life in some cultures.

It's time to shatter the stigma around women's sexuality.

Yes, progress has been made. But even modern women suffer in guilt, shame and fear of liberating their sexuality to enjoy true satisfaction and confidence.

That's why I believe that owning, enjoying, and even flaunting our divine right to enjoy sensual and sexual pleasure is the ultimate act of empowerment. Sex is the final frontier of women's empowerment, because our sexuality is taboo. For many women, it's hard to talk about and even harder to act on, if they do at all.

So when a woman embraces and celebrates her birthright to enjoy her body and all the glory of her six senses, and how it enhances every aspect of her life, she rejects society's conventions on the most intimate level, and that empowers her to create a life that sparkles—explodes!—with passion and purpose.

You can do that here in *The Biss Tribe: Where You Activate Your GoddessPleasure.*

Welcome to the place where you can flip the switch inside yourself to manifest the mind shifts, the lifestyle changes, the people, and the experiences that you need to maximize your infinite potential.

So please follow me through the GoddessPleasure Gateway into the life that you desire and deserve, and never look back.

How to Use This Book to Change Your Life

This book invites you to immerse in your imagination and embark on a week-long retreat among the 22 women who join The Biss Tribe on the mind- and life-shifting journey up Infinity Mountain.

Along the way, you will engage in discussions, activities, meditations and writing exercises that help you activate your GoddessPleasure.

To make this process simple for you, you'll find QR codes that will connect you with audio and video recordings for guided meditations, The GoddessPleasure Promise, and other helpful recitations.

You can also use the accompanying workbook, *PowerJournal to Activate Your GoddessPleasure,* available here:

Order Here

And you can take this experience to the next level by joining The Goddess RoundTable online community and by attending virtual and in-person GoddessPower Retreats led by me. Please learn more at TheGoddessPowerShow.com.

The secret to your success in The Biss Tribe is that you get out what you put in.

Remember, how you do anything is how you do everything. When you give it your all, you reap exponential rewards beyond your wildest dreams. On the contrary, mediocrity and half-assed efforts keep you stuck.

So, now it's time to invest your mind, body and spirit into this experience, and you will hardly recognize the woman you become, living the life that—until now—you've only dreamed about.

You can do it, Goddess, because *you* have the power!

I believe in you with infinite love,
Biss
Elizabeth Ann Atkins
Author & Creator of The Biss Tribe
Creator & Host of The GoddessPower Show®
with Elizabeth Ann Atkins
Co-Founder of
Two Sisters Writing & Publishing®

Contents

Welcome to The Biss Tribe: Where You
Activate Your GoddessPleasure vii

How to Use This Book to Change Your Life ix

Dedication & Acknowledgement xv

Your Itinerary for The Biss Tribe Retreat

Tuesday Day 3: Your GoddessPleasure Activation Begins

Ascending to The GoddessPleasure Tent 3

Treasure Chest Treats Help Awaken Kundalini Energy 16

The GoddessPleasure Promise 20

Brunch is Served: Feasting on Decadent Finger Foods . . .24

How Pleasure is the Portal to Your Power 32

Live Like Life is Making Love to You 40

Setting GoddessPleasure Intentions in
The Biss Tribe Class #88 50

Write Your GoddessPleasure Script. 53

Find Your Pleasure by Identifying
How You Feel Pleasureless. 59

Welcome to The Bliss Tribe

Your GoddessPleasure Awakening 61

Let's Step Through the GoddessPleasure Gateway 63

Activate Your GoddessPleasure with
Sensuous Movement 68

Let's Talk about Sacred Sexuality 69

Using the Five GoddessPleasure Activation Tools 75

Discovering Your GoddessPleasure in the
Divine Dimensions 84

A Healing Meditation to Release Shame, Guilt,
Fear and Trauma Around Your Sexuality 106

The Power of Pleasure: The Fifth GoddessPleasure
Activation Tool 127

Know Your Own Body First 133

Women's Pleasure Centers 101 134

Orgasms! 136

Explore & Enjoy Self-Pleasure! 144

Let's Close the Orgasm Gap 146

Sounding the Alarms in Your GoddessPleasure
Mission Control Center 153

Take a Refreshing Walk on the Pleasure Trail 155

Welcome to Your Personal GoddessPleasure Tent 156

The GoddessFeast on the Pleasure Tent Terrace 158

GoddessFeast Speaker: The Venus Roman Story 166

Discussing Aphrodisiacs in the Hot Springs 180

Time for Self-Exploration 186

Toy Time 187

Contents

Continue Your Transformation on Infinity Mountain 190

Stay Connected and Inspired in the Goddess
RoundTable Community 191

The Biss Tribe: Where You Celebrate
Your GoddessCoronation .193

Books in The Biss Tribe Series 193

Roster. 195
About the Author 203
Endnotes. 211

Dedication & Acknowledgement

The Biss Tribe: Where You Activate Your GoddessPleasure is dedicated to every person who was born into a female body and identity and has ever felt shamed, guilted, afraid or stifled around her divine birthright to enjoy the Pleasures of her mind, body and soul.

Thank you, Bastet, the Egyptian Goddess of Pleasure, and Aphrodite, the Greek Goddess of Pleasure, for inspiring us to courageously explore our wildest desires.

Your Itinerary for The Biss Tribe Retreat

Tuesday Day 3

Your Goddess Pleasure Activation Begins

Infinity Mountain

SeaGoddess Castle

The GoddessPeace Garden

The GoddessWarrior Fortress

The GoddessTreasure Cave

The GoddessPleasure Tent

The GoddessPower Pyramid

The Biss Tribe Retreat

The Biss Tribe Inn

© Elizabeth Ann Atkins 2024

Ascending to The Goddess Pleasure Tent

As the bus heads up the winding two-lane road on Infinity Mountain, you gaze through the window at the early-morning sunshine that's glowing on rugged rocks and boulders, lush green plants, bursts of orange flowers and huge trees.

To the left is a low metal rail at the edge of a steep drop-off that's so high, the treetops sway beneath it, above the vast valley where you arrived Sunday and stayed at The Biss Tribe Inn. To your right is a rugged wall of orange-beige striated rock which was blasted to make the road.

"We're going so high, my ears are popping!" Kiki exclaims as the 21 women around you, along with Biss and Esmerelda in the front seat, talk quietly, look out the windows and journal.

Kiki presses her hands to her ears. "It hurts. Maybe we're supposed to feel pain before we get to the Pleasure Tent. My kinda party."

"It's symbolic," Sunshine muses, "going way out of our comfort zones to go higher than we've ever been in life."

"Love that, sis," Jade says, glancing up from writing in her *PowerJournal*.

You're in an aisle seat beside Zeusse, who's nervously looking out the window. Wearing all black—loose trousers and a T-shirt made of soft, flowy cotton—she grips the arm rests.

"I might be tall, but I'm not a fan of heights," she says, looking pale as fear roils in her wide-set eyes. "My Pops took me to the Empire State Building once when I was ten years old, and I literally fainted. Two hours of this and five more days to come—my ass is *toast*."

Marla shoots up from her high-backed purple velvet seat in front of you and looks at Zeusse. "Just don't look down!"

"Easier said than done on this road, sweetheart," Zeusse says.

Marla tells you and Zeusse, "I don't know if I'm shaking from this ride, or from how scared I am to go to the Pleasure Tent."

"Face your fears, bitch!" Sammie says playfully beside her, shooting up to stand and rest her elbows around the headrest. "Marl, you're about to awaken your inner freak, and I'm about to lock mine in a room for a year."

They raise their hands and do the GoddessGreeting—a double high-five, followed by lacing their fingers together, over their heads, so they form a bridge—while saying in unison, "You can do it, Goddess, because *you* have the power!"

Then they laugh and hug, their long straight black and blond hair swirling together. Marla's brown sugar complexion and Sammie's vanilla-hued skin contrast as they flash big smiles with plump, glossed lips, never smudging their black-winged eyeliner and thick lashes.

"Did anyone notice we're twins today?" Sammie asks, shifting her shoulders to model the pink, form-fitting zip-front top with matching leggings that she and Marla are wearing.

"You're both adorable," Sunshine says. "Hashtag BFF goals."

"Good one, mama!" Marla says, doing the GoddessGreeting over the aisle with Sunshine.

You shift in your chair, feeling so comfortable in the clothes that you put on this morning in your room at the GoddessPower Pyramid. You and all the women are wearing styles that reflect your personalities—leggings and form-fitting tank tops, loose trousers and T-shirts, flowy linen pants and tunics, and loafers,

Tuesday, Day 3

sandals and athletic shoes—all in shades of pink, purple, gold and black.

You finger the black, egg-shaped crystal hanging on your necklace of luminescent white moonstone crystals, remembering how Biss said the black tourmaline blocks negative energy and the moonstones help activate your GoddessPower and figure out your life's path and purpose. You pinch the charms that jingle on the pendant and look at them: the Biss Tribe logo and the starburst inscribed with your name. You look around, noticing that every woman is wearing her necklace.

Across the aisle, Jade stops writing in her *PowerJournal* and runs her fingertips over the colorful goddesses and vines tattooed on her arms. Peace radiates from her hazel eyes and round face as she says, "I don't know about any of you, but I actually feel better than I've felt in a very long time."

"As do I," Delaney adds with a nod that makes her silver curls bounce over her shoulders. "But will it last? Can we sustain this feeling when we get back home?"

"I wonder that, too, sis, because I'm scared of myself," Jade confesses, using a scrunchie to put her pink hair into a ponytail. "I am so lazy sometimes! I just have to keep envisioning myself traveling the world with my band and leaving my old, stifling life behind."

Marla turns around and offers Jade the GoddessGreeting.

"Now my ears are really popping!" Jade says as the bus heads up a steep incline. "Ouch!"

As you look out the window, a speeding truck suddenly veers around a sharp curve, coming straight at the bus.

The women shriek.

"Aw, snap!" Zeusse exclaims.

Welcome to The Biss Tribe

The bus swerves onto the narrow shoulder. You sway and grip your seat.

Crunch! The wheels grind over gravel.

"Lord help us!" Celeste cries out as the bus zigzags.

"OhmyGod!" Marla screams as the jagged wall of rock appears inches outside the bus window. "Don't crash!"

She and Sammie grip the headrests, then drop to their seats.

"Holy shit, man!" Andi says. "We almost got smashed like a bug against the rocks! And that little guard rail is all that's separating us from plunging down into—"

"Don't say that!" Sunshine snips. "Biss says our words create our reality. So I'm declaring that we're safely getting to the Pleasure Tent."

"True that," Zeusse groans.

"Don't worry, Goddesses!" the bus driver, Vee, says over the loudspeaker, as the bus returns to the pavement and stabilizes. "I got you. We'll be arriving at The GoddessPleasure Tent shortly."

Biss stands to face you and the women. "My Goddesses! You all okay? Let this serve as a reminder that when you activate your GoddessPower, it fortifies a supernatural forcefield of protection around you, 24/7. Know that. And I can't wait for you to see the tantalizing treats at The GoddessPleasure Tent."

"That's what's up," Zeusse says softly as Biss sits down. "Can't get there soon enough." She pulls her long dreads over one shoulder, then pulls out her journal and begins writing with an intense expression, becoming oblivious to the chatter around you.

You look down at yours, pinching the tiny metal lightning bolt and the Biss Tribe logo charms, then run your fingertips over the citrine crystal bracelet on the same wrist.

"I hope that near-miss wasn't a bad omen for things to come," Kiki says.

Tuesday, Day 3

"Right," Bianca says, glancing back nervously. "This is triggering my PTSD from the crash." She closes her eyes and takes deep breaths. "Plus that big black SUV behind us that's full of security guards is a reminder of all the forces just waiting to pounce on us to stop us from doing everything we came here to achieve—"

"That scares the fuck outta me," Andi says.

Sammie stands up again, her blue eyes roiling with anxiety as she glosses her pink lips with a gold tube. "Yeah, I'm so scared that my old mindset and lifestyle will pull me back into temptation with men. Even though it sucked! I really want to believe that my vision during meditation yesterday can be my new life with my dream husband."

"And that our skincare line," Marla chimes in, "is a huge success."

"Yeah," Sammie says, "like eight-figure boss bitches rockin' the world."

Kiki sighs. "Sammie, you're so lucky you found your purpose in life. I hope mine shows up on this freaking mountain. But Andi, I'm with you on the security guards. That's scary as shit. Like, what if the threat here is much worse than they're telling us?"

Several women groan. A worried murmur erupts in the seats around you.

"Welcome to The GoddessPleasure Tent," Esmerelda announces, standing at the front of the bus and facing the women. Ornate golden gates open to reveal a gold-brick driveway lined with bursts of purple flowers, tall trees and green grass.

"Wow!" Bianca exclaims as women gasp.

"OhmyGod!" Marla sighs. "How can I *not* take pics and vids there?"

"That tent is breathtaking!" Sunshine says.

Welcome to The Biss Tribe

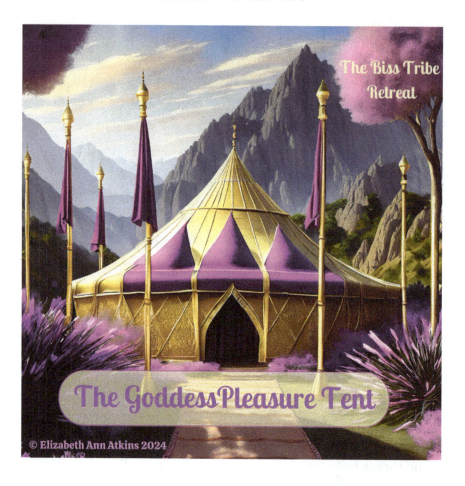

The huge tent is made of thick gold fabric with purple accents. The Biss Tribe flag flies on a tall pole at the center.

"This reminds me," Delaney says, "of a film featuring Arabian knights who stop at an exotic desert oasis, where luscious delights await those fortunate enough to enter."

"This is a film featuring Goddesses," Kiki says, playfully flipping her platinum-tipped brunette hair as her dark eyes sparkle, "about to make our fantasies come true."

As the bus gets closer, you see that purple velvet curtains adorned with sparkling crystals drape the entrance.

"Is this real?" Jade gasps.

Tuesday, Day 3

"Yes, it's very real," Esmerelda says. "Ladies, get ready for a sensory extravaganza that will awaken your mind, body and spirit to a new way of experiencing life. You will *never* be the same after your stay here."

Biss rises from the front seat and holds up a *PowerJournal*. "My gorgeous Goddesses, please write as much as possible to record your thoughts, feelings and revelations during this experience. We're tailoring everything—your food, drinks, clothing, activities and accommodations—to enhance your experience, so that you can curate your GoddessPleasure lifestyle back home. Everybody repeat after me: I deserve to activate my GoddessPleasure!"

You and the women repeat that in unison.

"One more time!" Biss orders as Vee parks the bus.

"I deserve to activate my GoddessPleasure!" you all exclaim.

"That means," Biss says, "you will incorporate Pleasure into every aspect of living. And you won't believe how luscious your life will become."

"Yes!" Celeste's big brown eyes sparkle and her golden molasses-hued complexion glows with excitement. "I am so ready for that! Watch me go from stressed-out CEO with itching, bleeding eczema, to a baking Goddess who's getting her Pleasure and serving it up to folks in my cakes and pies."

Biss beams at Celeste and says, "There you go, Goddess!"

Andi grumbles, "I guess this means I have to stop eating a bologna sandwich with chips on a paper plate for dinner, and treat myself to my favorite tacos and burritos—"

"Every damn day, girlfriend!" Celeste says, offering Andi the GoddessGreeting as they say, "You can do it, Goddess, because *you* have the power!"

"Live like the divine royalty that you are!" Sunshine adds. "No more saving the best clothes or food or dishes for a special occasion."

Welcome to The Biss Tribe

"I want to make every minute feel like a special occasion," Bianca adds. "Life is short."

"Yes!" Biss says. "Spoil yourselves! Show the world how you demand to be treated, lavished with royal treatment, and people will respond accordingly."

"Look," Marla whispers, staring out the window. The security guards are standing in front of the tent, flanking each side of the purple-carpeted walkway that leads to the entrance.

Sammie's eyes grow wide. "What the—"

"Are there like, people hiding in the bushes?" Jade asks.

"Biss, are we safe?" Andi asks. "Why all the security?"

"As I said at The Biss Tribe Inn," Biss says, "that group called BRUTE wants to stop us. They are foot soldiers of global patriarchal dominance. And since the co-founder of Husbands, Incorporated, Venus Roman will be our speaker tonight at The GoddessFeast, we need extra security today. Please just relax and know that you are safe."

Zeusse purses her lips and casts a pessimistic look at the guards. "Snap. Where there's smoke, there's fire."

Several women whisper to each other in worrisome tones.

"Ladies, it's time to enter The GoddessPleasure tent," Esmerelda says with a smile. "Your Concierges will guide you inside, first to the restroom, then to your seats. After the day's activities, you'll be guided to your private tents to prepare for the GoddessFeast and festivities."

The bus doors open, and you join the women filing out, onto the carpeted walk. A Concierge on each side of the entrance pulls a satin rope that makes the velvet drapes dramatically flutter open.

Exotic music with drumming, exotic chimes and a woman's satiny, sultry, wordless song welcome you inside. You close your eyes to savor the scent of jasmine and aromatic food.

"Mmmmmmm," Sunshine says, "that scent is heavenly!"

Tuesday, Day 3

You're in a vestibule whose every surface is covered with drapey satin, tassels and glitter amidst ornate fountains, trees and plants that sparkle with tiny white and purple lights. You can't see where the music and scents are coming from, but Biss and Esmerelda are standing in front of an interior entryway that's covered by layers of gold, magenta, and purple satin drapes and flanked by lighted trees.

"Ladies," Esmerelda says, raising her arms to the left and right. "Please make your way to the restrooms on either side of the lobby, then we'll assemble here and enter your GoddessPleasure Activation Station."

A short time later, as you gather with all the women, Biss and Esmerelda step to the sides of the entryway. The drapes open to reveal a huge space that glows with pink, purple and gold lights. The delicious food scents waft even stronger, and the music is louder.

"My Goddesses," Biss says, beaming, "Welcome to The GoddessPleasure Tent!"

You and all the women step past Biss and Esmerelda into the huge tent whose ceilings and walls are draped with swaths of jewel-toned satin that extend from the round sides of the tent and extend up to the top of a golden pole at its center.

Bianca maneuvers her power chair and gazes up in awe at the Moroccan-style metal lanterns that hang throughout the tent and cast stencil-like patterns on the walls, the ceiling, and the scene below.

"Wow, this tent is an amphitheater!" Jade exclaims, as you and the women stand in a large space at the top of a wide, carpeted staircase. It leads down three wide tiers that descend in a half-circle to a sunken, circular stage. Each tier holds eight loveseat-sized, legless sofas that are low and plush velvet, cushioned with fancy pillows, draped with faux-fur blankets and set in wooden arms and backs that are carved with cherubs and hearts.

In front of each sofa is a low rectangular table made of the same carved wood as the sofas, which are black, indigo, magenta, emerald green and burnt orange. Each woman's Treasure Chest already sits on the tables, along with tissues protruding from decorative covers made of tiny, colorful glass squares that glisten in the shifting light.

"Oh, my goodness," Sunshine gasps, "I don't know where to look first."

"Spectacular!" Delaney says with awe. "My heart is pounding."

"This is a trip," Zeusse adds.

"It's so romantic," Sammie sighs.

"And sexy," Celeste says. "Makes me feel a certain way—"

The music blasts and dozens of dancers—male and female in every human hue—twirl out seemingly from nowhere, surrounding you and the women. They're dazzling in costumes that jingle with gold coins, finger symbols and glittery fabrics showcasing the dancers's beautiful bodies.

You and the women watch in awe as the men's bare, chiseled chests and broad, muscled shoulders glimmer as if lightly oiled. Gold, silver and copper belts cinch their waists and support Egyptian-style man-skirts, exposing powerful thigh muscles that flex as they dance. Their black-lined eyes cast sultry passion as they lock into your gaze as if you're the most mesmerizing woman they've ever seen.

The women do the same, like a troupe of twirling genies who are ready to grant your every wish, while their eyes sparkle with fierce, fiery passion.

"I want *that* look in my eyes," Jade says loudly, close to your ear.

The female dancers flip their heads—some flowing with long hair of all colors—others bald, braided, afroed or adorned with

Tuesday, Day 3

bouncy bobs, twists and dreads. Their sparkling costumes showcase voluptuous breasts and hourglass shapes in belly-baring skirts banded with jewels set in gold and holding up sheer, floaty fabrics that reveal toned legs. The liquid movements of the women's shoulders, arms, hands and fingers are so smooth, they seem to defy human anatomy.

"Am I dreaming?" Zeusse asks loudly as the dancers shimmy and jingle around each woman.

"I hope not!" Celeste says as the Concierges begin to guide each of you to your personal plush sofas.

The music softens as the dancers descend stairs on each side of the amphitheater, and gather on the stage around Biss.

"Ladies, please get comfortable," Esmerelda says. "Keep your *PowerJournals* handy to record any ideas that come to mind."

A Concierge carries Bianca to her sofa near you on the top tier in the center, which provides a sweeping view of all the women settling amidst plush pillows on the low sofas. At the same time, the dancers twirl on the sunken stage in a synchronized dance—creating a human kaleidoscope—as their colorful, bejeweled costumes dazzle in a symmetrical shimmer.

"My Goddesses!" exclaims Biss, who's wearing a curve-hugging, cream-colored, sparkly lace dress with drapey sleeves and mermaid-esque ruffles at the knees. She raises her arms toward the dancers. "It's time for more Pleasure in your life!"

"Yes," the women cheer.

The Concierges bring you and every woman a small, bejeweled tray offering a personalized assortment of flat or sparkling water in a gold goblet and a pot of coffee or tea with a pretty China cup and saucer, plus honey, cream and sugar. Pouring and clinking sounds, along with the scent of coffee and peppermint tea, fill the air as you and the women enjoy the beverages.

Welcome to The Biss Tribe

"Here at The GoddessPleasure Tent," Biss says, "we're shifting into a new vortex where every moment of every day and night, we seek Pleasure in what we see, feel, touch, taste, smell, hear and experience through our five physical senses and our intuition, our Supernatural Selves, which connect us to the infinite, divine energy of the universe."

A screen drops above and behind Biss as the dancers twirl around her and sultry Arabian music plays.

"So what exactly is GoddessPleasure?" Biss asks as a graphic appears on the screen.

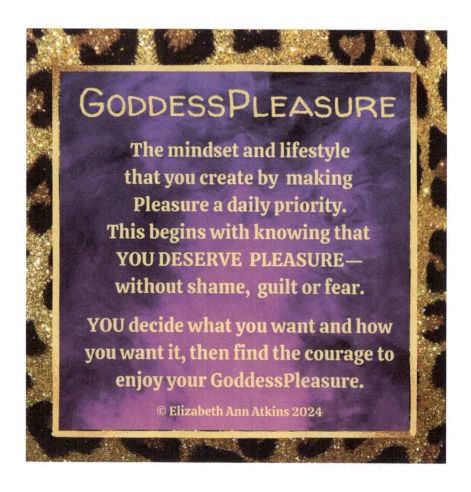

GoddessPleasure

The mindset and lifestyle that you create by making Pleasure a daily priority. This begins with knowing that YOU DESERVE PLEASURE— without shame, guilt or fear.

YOU decide what you want and how you want it, then find the courage to enjoy your GoddessPleasure.

© Elizabeth Ann Atkins 2024

Tuesday, Day 3

"GoddessPleasure," Biss says, "is the mindset and lifestyle that you create by making Pleasure a daily priority. This begins with knowing that YOU DESERVE PLEASURE—without shame, guilt or fear. YOU decide what you want and how you want it, then find the courage to enjoy your GoddessPleasure."

Seated beside you, Sunshine looks worried. "I want to embrace all of this, but something inside me feels *so* guilty. Like a bad girl. That's what Nani and my aunt always told me. Even when I hear the word 'Pleasure,' I feel like a bad girl who'll get punished for wanting it and doing anything about it."

Marla, who's sitting in front of you next to Sammie, turns around and nods. "That's like, exactly my story."

"And the opposite of mine!" Sammie says playfully.

"Today will relieve of you of Good Girl Syndrome," Biss says. "I want you to step away from here knowing that Pleasure is not bad. It's a gift that you receive when you're born into a female body. And I want you to know that your GoddessPleasure is not all about sex. It's anything that excites your senses and makes you happy."

"Pleasure is a tactile experience," Biss says, tickling her fingers through the air. "Run your fingers over the velvet sofa. Touch the satiny tassels on the pillows. Inhale and savor the scent of your coffee or tea, and the spicy smells of brunch that's coming soon. Let the music sweep you away. Focus on the beautiful scenery. And acknowledge the joy in your spirit that your GoddessLife is yours for the taking."

Several women close their eyes and smile slightly, but others look sullen.

"This is all well and good," Bianca says, "but back in my reality, I get so stressed and overwhelmed. I don't know if I can—"

"You can!" Biss shouts. "Bianca, and all of you, you absolutely *can* do this! Everybody say, 'I *can* create my GoddessLife with lots of Pleasure!'"

The women repeat that in unison.

Treasure Chest Treats Help Awaken Kundalini Energy

As the dancers slowly move around Biss, she says, "Open your Treasure Chests, and go to the Pleasure compartment."

There you find a bracelet made of red and orange crystal beads, along with a red crystal heart charm, a bottle of rose oil, a small candle and a scroll.

Excited chatter ripples through the tent as the women discover today's treasures. Concierge Jami appears and attaches the heart to your bracelet, which amplifies the jingles as the women put on and shake their crystal bracelets.

"These red and orange carnelian beads," Biss says, "raise your vibrational frequency and help balance and activate the two lower chakras—the root and the sacral—which are all about sexual health, creativity and sensual Pleasure. That's also where our Kundalini energy awaits activation to help our GoddessPleasure blaze."

"Our Kunda-what?" Andi asks.

The screen behind Biss shows the silhouette of a woman with a coil of golden energy around her tailbone.

"Kundalini energy," Biss says, "is our life force. It's a form of our divine feminine energy and it's an integral part of our GoddessPower, and our GoddessPleasure."

On the screen, the red root chakra and the orange sacral chakra glow in the gold mist at the base of the spine in the female silhouette.

Tuesday, Day 3

"Our Kundalini energy resides at the base of the spine," Biss says, "in and around our root and sacral chakras, and it helps awaken our creativity and our Supernatural Selves."

The definition of Supernatural Self appears on the screen. "You remember what you learned Sunday at The Biss Tribe Inn," Biss says. "That your Supernatural Self is the Goddess version of you who's led by your Spirit and is fueled and informed by the currents of power pulsing in and around you from the universal field of knowledge. This supernatural energy amplifies your truth, guides your every thought and action, and synchronizes your manifestations and life mission."

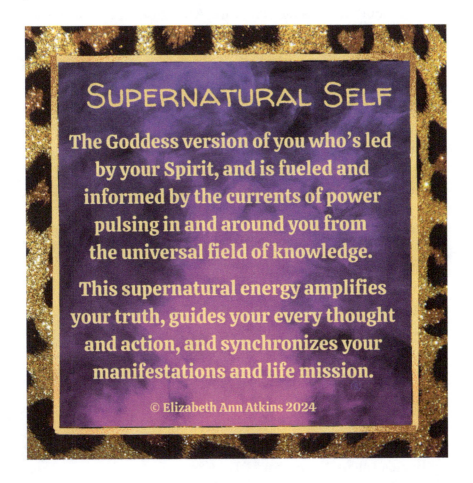

Welcome to The Biss Tribe

The word "kundalini" appears on the screen above the female silhouette.

"This ancient concept of Kundalini energy is rooted in Hinduism and Tantric yoga," Biss says, as "kundal" and "ini" show up on the screen. "'Kundal' means 'coils' and 'ini' means 'power.' You can imagine it coiled around the base of your spine like a snake."

The gold mist begins to swirl and rise as each chakra lights up, finally illuminating the lavender crown chakra.

"Our goal is to awaken our Kundalini energy," Biss says.

Kiki raises a hand. "How do we do that?"

"With our five GoddessPleasure Activation Tools," Biss says, "Pranayama breathing, chakra clearing, meditation and journaling, plus one very juicy one that I'll share later." Biss flashes a big smile. "Now, back to your Treasure Chest treats. The symbolism of the red heart speaks for itself here in The GoddessPleasure Tent. Now open the bottle of rose oil, which has the highest vibrational frequency of all essential oils."

You pull out the little bottle.

"Put a drop on your palms," Biss says. "Rub it together, cup your hands over your nose, and inhale."

A Concierge hands Biss a bottle and she demonstrates as you and the women do the same.

"Mmmmmm," Biss says, echoing a chorus of delighted moans from the women.

"This is heavenly," Sunshine says, repeatedly inhaling the scent from her palms that are cupped around her nose.

"I loooooove it," Jade says, closing her eyes. "I must write a song. I'll call it Healing My Kundalini Rose."

Andi smiles. "Sounds like a theme song for today, and the hidden meaning isn't lost on me."

Bianca smiles. "Love that."

Tuesday, Day 3

"That's clever, Jade," Biss says. "Blooming roses, of course, are very yonic."

"What's yonic?" Kiki asks.

"You've heard of phallic, which means shaped like a penis," Biss says. "Yonic comes from Yoni, which symbolizes the Hindu goddess Shakti. She embodies power, energy and the divine feminine. So Yonic is a Sanskrit word for something that looks like female genitalia—"

"Like orchids," Zeusse says, holding the bottle to her nose. "Yo, I'm not into perfume, but this is about to be my go-to secret to zen out. Biss, can a female wear essential oil as her perfume?"

Biss nods. "You can dab it on pulse points, and put it in your hair. It's very concentrated, so it's best to dilute it with a carrier oil like coconut oil. Or you can put it in a spray bottle with distilled water and spray it onto your clothes or in a room."

Biss smiles. "One more thing, the scent of roses is scientifically shown to stimulate arousal and boost your sex drive, for men and women."

Zeusse holds up the bottle. "Rose oil. That'll be my first gift to my next boo."

"Aphrodisiac" appears on the screen.

"My Goddesses," Biss says, "this word is a major theme here at The GoddessPleasure Tent. The word aphrodisiac comes from the ancient Greek goddess of love, Aphrodite. As you know, an aphrodisiac is anything that you eat, drink, smell, see, feel or otherwise experience that stimulates your sexual desire. They enhance your GoddessPleasure, so you're going to learn how to incorporate them into your GoddessLife back home."

Biss inhales the rose oil from her palms. "This divine scent is an aphrodisiac in a lot of cultures because it stimulates your Pleasure centers. Plus, it calms you and boosts your confidence."

Video on the screen shows tight red and pink rose buds exploding into glorious blooms.

"And very importantly," Biss says, "rose oil helps with healing, and today we'll be healing wounds around Pleasure. Specifically, the shame, guilt and fear that society, families and religion impose on girls and women to control us into conforming to their oppressive and damaging rules around sensuality and sexuality."

"I'm the queen of *that,* unfortunately," Marla announces as Sammie, in the sofa beside her, nods.

"We all are," Sunshine adds.

"I fucking hate that," Andi groans. "It's so unfair."

"This bitch is about to be free!" Marla exclaims.

"That's what's up," Zeusse says.

"With rose oil and all the essential oils that we use here in The Biss Tribe," Biss says, "one whiff can push your reset button and elevate you back into your GoddessPleasure Zone."

"Let's go!" Celeste says.

The GoddessPleasure Promise

Biss raises a scroll tied with a purple satin ribbon as the dancers gently swirl around her. "My Goddesses, get the scroll from the Pleasure section in your Treasure Chest."

You reach into your Treasure Chest and retrieve the papyrus-like paper that crackles as you and the women untie the ribbons and unroll the scrolls.

"Recite this with me," Biss says. "This will be your daily recitation from now on... to reprogram your brain to know that you deserve Pleasure every day. It will help you release any stigma and shame around your sexuality, and it will free you to experience your life's wildest desires."

Tuesday, Day 3

Marla raises her hand. "Do we have to say this *and* The GoddessPower Promise every day?"

"Yes," Biss says. "There's a special GoddessPromise for Power, Pleasure, Prosperity, Protection and Peace. You'll learn a new one at each Activation Station. Then when you go home, you'll say the entire Promise every morning and evening."

"That's a lot!" Sammie says, holding a steaming teacup.

"What you want is a lot," Biss snaps, "and this is how you make it happen. Who's *not* willing to put in the work?"

Nobody raises her hand.

"That's what I thought! And as I said, you'll record your GoddessPower Promise in the studios at SeaGoddess Castle, so you can listen to your own voice reciting this, morning and night. Got it?"

"One thousand percent," Zeusse says.

Sunshine nods. "That's the power of Autosuggestion, like Napoleon Hill says in *Think and Grow Rich*, right Biss?"

"Exactly," she says. "I used this technique to lose 100 pounds and get super fit, power through a terrible divorce to make healing miracles and harmony happen, and to achieve so many other things that had once seemed impossible."

"Sounds worth the work to me," Bianca says.

Biss leads you and the women to recite in unison The GoddessPleasure Promise:

The GoddessPleasure Promise

Pleasure is the portal to my power, so I cultivate Pleasure in everything I do, all day and night.

I courageously and shamelessly embrace my divine right to enjoy the sensual Pleasures of life in ways that are safe and serve my highest good. I have zero guilt or shame about pleasuring myself and enjoying the thrills of my own body, and I enjoy exploring new ways to delight myself, with or without a partner or other people.

I know that orgasms are an important part of my wellness, as they are proven in research to improve my mood, my immune system, my self-esteem and my confidence, while helping me sleep, promoting longevity, making me glow from the inside out, and releasing oxytocin, the Pleasure hormone, which is the antidote to cortisol, the stress hormone that causes inflammation, early aging and illness.

I know that my Pleasure is my responsibility, and that the mind is the sexiest organ in the body. I devote time each day to affirming my divine birthright to enjoy the sensual Pleasures of my body.

I release all shame, guilt and fear around my sexuality, and I commit to a daily practice that reminds me that I deserve to indulge the sensual thrills of my mind, body and spirit. I always practice safety first as I reject the rules imposed by society, religion and families that rob girls and women of physical Pleasure. I know that I have the Power to explore new ways of living and loving, and to design my own lovestyle and lifestyle accordingly.

When I'm with a partner, I have the courage to speak up to set and enforce my boundaries of what I will and will not do. My personal empire welcomes those who honor my boundaries, while expelling and repelling those intending to disregard and disrespect me.

Tuesday, Day 3

Every choice that I make throughout the day and night is motivated by the question, "How can I do this in a way that will bring me the greatest Pleasure?" Because when I enjoy something, I do it better, and this creates more magical moments that all add up to my life.

I pursue Pleasure in every act of living, including the smallest moments of: eating; drinking; sleeping; touching a soft surface; inhaling fresh air; feeling the sunshine on my face; smelling a flower; hearing a loved one's voice; laughing; moving my body; enjoying the company, comfort and love of my family and friends; experiencing water in the shower, bath, pool, or sea; and engaging in the activities that bring me joy. I practice tantric living, which means fusing the power of mind, body and spirit into every moment to create a mindfulness that multiplies Pleasure on every level.

I know that Pleasure is my divine birthright as a Goddess. I claim it. I believe it. I know it. I live it. Because I am infinite and unstoppable in my GoddessPleasure.

Welcome to The Biss Tribe

Dear Goddess Reader, you can listen to Biss reciting The GoddessPleasure Promise by using this QR code.

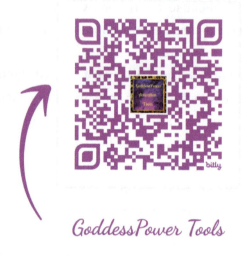

GoddessPower Tools

Brunch is Served: Feasting on Decadent Finger Foods

As you and the women return your scrolls to your Treasure Chests, your Concierges appear in the aisles, carrying large silver platters that send delicious food scents wafting through the air.

"Holy moley." Andi tilts her head back, closing her eyes and inhaling deeply. "I'm drooling for whatever that is! Man!"

"Let your mouths water for the decadent GoddessFeast that's coming now," Biss says. "This is a brunch like you've never experienced."

Concierge Jami brings you a large silver tray filled with your favorite finger foods artistically arranged in exotic leaves and edible flowers. They also serve a silver challis of your favorite beverage.

Tuesday, Day 3

Each woman receives a similar tray on her table; many slip into loungey positions—stretching out along the length of the sofa or lying on their sides, all with their lavish platters within easy reach.

"My beautiful Goddesses," Biss says, "before you take a bite, let's close our eyes and give thanks to the infinite, divine powers for gifting us with this experience and this nourishment that fuels our minds, bodies and souls to activate our GoddessPleasure here in the Pleasure Tent, so that we can create luscious lives that delight us and illuminate the world. And so it is spoken, and so it is done."

You and the women repeat a deep chorus of: "And so it is spoken, and so it is done."

From the side of the stage, Esmerelda announces, "Please also know that no one here has a nut allergy, so you're safe to enjoy them if they're part of your feast."

You savor the food that's far more delicious than you remember it being back in your regular life.

"Oh. My. Goddess!" Marla exclaims, closing her eyes and moaning with the first bite. "How can this taste *soooo* good?"

"What do you have?" Sammie asks.

"The Middle Eastern feast," Marla says, dipping a stuffed grape leaf into baba ghanoush, then wrapping her lips around it, closing her eyes and moaning again. She gazes at the skewered mini-kabobs of shrimp and chicken with grilled veggies, hummus, tabouli and baklava.

Sammie points to her platter that holds a pretty arrangement of cheeses, meats, fruit, nuts, bread sticks and chocolates—all adorned with edible flowers. "This is the most beautiful and delicious charcuterie board I've ever seen. I am on Cloud Nine right now."

Beside you, Sunshine uses a tiny fork to lift an escargot from golden puff pastry and garlic butter. She says, "They know me too well! Blue cheese-crusted steak bites. Truffle fries. Brussel sprouts. And mini cheesecakes! I am just *done!*"

Delaney, holding chop sticks to sample from her tray of colorful sushi on tropical leaves, nods with an ecstatic expression.

The food, drink, dancers and décor—amidst the music and perfumed air—are intoxicating.

From the stage, Biss has an amused expression as she watches all of you indulge. "My Goddesses! Take a mental snapshot of this moment so you can write about it later in your *PowerJournal*. Listen to the music and feel it beating in rhythm with your heart. Inhale the scents rising from your platters. Visually devour the artistic arrangements of your food. Savor the flavors while you stay mindful and present in this magic moment to maximize the bliss of every bite and sip."

She speaks in a sultry tone: "Feast your eyes on the spectacular scene around you. Caress the fabrics. Deeply feel the joy of your spirit as she—the real you who's awakening to your greatest GoddessPleasure here in The Biss Tribe—is showing you, telling you, how she wants to feel, all day, every day, for the rest of your life. Pampered. Loving life. Enjoying the thrill of all your senses coming alive. Know that you can create these feelings back at home, and settle for nothing less. This is GoddessPleasure Life!"

The music intensifies and the dancers become more frenzied in formation around Biss. They're like a flower opening around her, as she stands at the center. The dancers shimmy and gyrate and burst up and out in unison, and you can't look away.

"Savor this moment," Biss commands, "with all your senses! Allow the Pleasure of what you see, taste, hear, touch, smell and sense in your spirit to become so overwhelming, that you have a life-gasm."

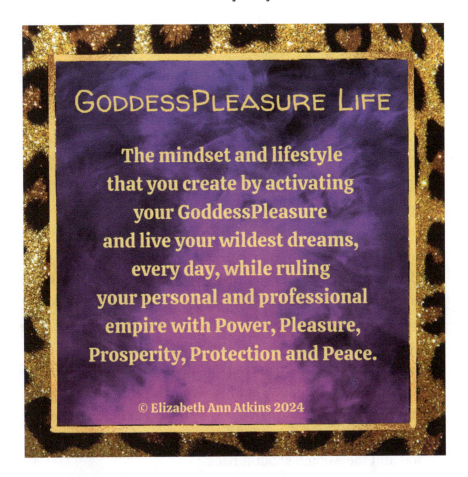

"What's that?" Andi asks, holding a taco close to her mouth.

"It's a moment that feels so overwhelmingly good, your body tingles and it feels as good as sex," Biss says. "You can have a life-gasm in a split-second moment of intense gratitude and relief, when tasting delicious food, when everything around you is synchronizing to create an unforgettable moment, and when you do something that makes you feel like a Bad Ass. Aim to fill your days with life-gasms!"

Jade shrieks. "Oh, *hell yeah!*"

Sunshine says, "Oh my God, a life-gasm! Who says that!?"

"Us, bitches!" Sammie roars. "We say that now! And we have them. A lot!"

"I like that," Zeusse says before biting into a lamb chop dipped in spicy sauce.

Sunshine wipes her mouth with a linen napkin and says: "Biss, I feel like such a bad girl because I want all of this and more! I love this feeling! But my whole body is burning with guilt and shame and fear."

"Yeah, like bad girl vibes," Marla says.

Biss looks up at Sunshine, then Marla, you and the other women.

"The fear, shame and guilt are real," Biss says. "Here is the place where we release it! Be gentle with yourself. And be patient. A lifetime of brainwashing doesn't just dissolve in an instant. It's a process. And I promise you, you can do it, starting here and now."

You can feel the electricity crackling in the air amidst the 22 women as you all process what Biss is saying and savor the decadent platters of food washed down by drinks in gold challises.

"Say 'life-gasm!'" Biss shouts.

You and the women shout it back.

"Louder!" Biss commands, "like you know you deserve it!"

"Life-gasm!" the women nearly scream.

"Yes!" Biss cheers. "You're going to leave here with the ability to suck pure Pleasure out of every experience. No more living and working in a numb fog of detachment. Feeling like life has put you on punishment. Or that you're watching life fly by while you feel unfulfilled and unsatisfied. No more depriving yourself of the Pleasures that are yours for the taking, but lie dormant under the awful weight of worries, regret, guilt, shame and fear! No more!"

The dancers curl down around Biss, like giant human beads that sparkle as they breathe, causing sweat on their backs, and jewels on their costumes, to move and reflect the colorful light.

Tuesday, Day 3

"It's time!" Biss shouts. "It's **TIME** for YOU, Goddess, to awaken to the magic of life. To find your Power in your Pleasure, because it recalibrates your mind, body and soul to activate energy you didn't know you had. And that infinite energy becomes the source of everything you need to create and rule your empire, however that looks for you."

Biss raises her hands, balls her fists, then flicks out all her fingers, so they stretch up and out. Her palms face you—like she's casting energy outward, directly at you and each woman.

"Take this electricity, this Goddess energy that's electrifying the air around us," Biss commands as the dancers crouch at her hips, moving in a circle as if she's standing in the eye of a human hurricane.

"Feel this energy pulse through you like an electric current that will power your mission, your dreams and the life you came here to create. Think about **your** definition of a life-gasm. You have the power to define what overwhelms you with emotional, physical and spiritual Pleasure, so you can experience limitless life-gasms during the day. This is your reality when you awaken to the Power of Pleasure as you've never known.

"Pleasure!" she shouts, as the dancers shoot up around her, their arms and fingers moving like a starburst. They crouch down.

"Power!" she exclaims. They shoot up again, then go down.

"Life-gasms!" she shouts as the dancers explode in a dizzying swirl, their sweat-sheened arms, fingers and faces glowing under the jewel-toned light from the lanterns above. "Pleasure is the portal to your Power, ladies. So let's learn how to use it!"

A few rows down, Celeste raises her arms in the air and tosses back her head. "I'm ready!" she shouts. "I am so ready!"

"My entire being feels more alive than I can remember," Jade says. "Like I could make a lightbulb glow if I touch it with my fingertip."

Welcome to The Biss Tribe

"Close your eyes," Biss says softly as the dancers sway around her. "Project this exhilarating energy onto the movie screen of your imagination, and envision how you can take what you're feeling now back home into your daily life while you build your empire."

The dancers sway around her like a soft wave.

"Envision yourself in the midst of your GoddessPleasure Life, experiencing Pleasure on every level, in vivid detail, with this magical energy twirling around everything you created, feeling the thrill of it in life-gasm after life-gasm."

All around you, the women are eating, captivated.

"Now in your *PowerJournal for Pleasure* section, write everything that you see and feel in that scene from your Goddess Vision, as it relates to Pleasure. Describe every aspect of Pleasure—in your mind, in your body and in your soul—that you feel while envisioning the new you, your new life, your new empire—as if it's real, now, in your 3-D physical experience every day. Write in a spirit of deep believing, *knowing,* that this is possible for you."

A few women groan.

"Easier said than done," Andi quips.

"I hear you." Biss has a compassionate tone. "There have been times when I was too depressed and discouraged to even pray. I just had to press through. But I didn't give up, and somewhere deep down, I knew that God/Spirit/Universe had given me this unstoppable GoddessPleasure to help me succeed."

Jade lets out a soft sob. "This is so hard. When I get 100 with myself, I'm legit in that spot. No hope. Depressed. Discouraged. Don't see a way out."

Biss presses praying hands to her chest and closes her eyes for a moment.

"This is your way out," she says, casting a soft gaze at Jade, then you, and everyone. "And if you don't believe it yet, then use

Tuesday, Day 3

your imagination. Like when you were a little girl playing dress-up, when you believed in the magic that anything is possible. Because when you activate your GoddessPleasure, anything *is* possible."

You listen and try to make your mind go there.

Jade speaks with a tinge of aggravation: "You're making it sound like Pleasure is more important than Power. It seems like Power would be the most important."

Biss nods. "That's totally correct, Jade. However, if our ability to enjoy Pleasure is stifled by conditioning from our families, religion and society, then we are not fully in our Power. We have to unleash our GoddessPleasure with gusto, in order to activate our greatest GoddessPower."

"That's what's up!" Zeusse says, sitting in a corner of her sofa with her long legs outstretched on the plush cushion. "I grew up with so much of that from my grandmother. Mama G went to church every day. And me being different—I knew I liked girls since kindergarten—she spoke all that Biblical shame over me every summer in Alabama. For a long time, I thought I really was a deviant like she said."

Zeusse covers her sad face with her hands for a moment. Then she lowers them, and a happier expression makes her smooth, coffee bean-brown complexion glow. "But fortunately, back in New York, my Pops let me know that God made me perfect just as I am. He took me to a progressive church where I met other kids like me. And he told his mother to stop criticizing me. Mama G did stop the words, but she could cut her eyes at me in a way that hurt my heart. That just made me more determined to love on females and enjoy Pleasure my own way."

"Zeusse," Biss says, "thank you for sharing how you transformed pain into power to live and love as you truly desire."

How Pleasure is the Portal to Your Power

The logo for The Goddess Power Show with Elizabeth Ann Atkins appears on the screen.

"For those of you who listen to my podcast," Biss says as the dancers sway around her, "you know that my mission is to explore taboo topics that help you live bigger, better and bolder to manifest your heart's wildest desires. These taboo topics often center around sexuality, because for women, that is the ultimate taboo."

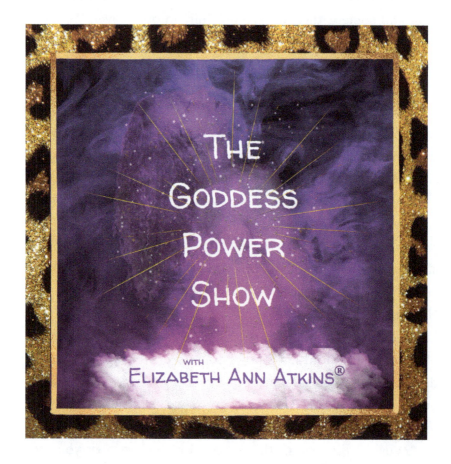

"That's why I interview guests who include experts and everyday people who are blazing new trails to think, act, live, love, work and play in ways that defy convention and ignite bliss."

Tuesday, Day 3

Marla moans. "This baklava is bliss. The best I've ever had."

Zeusse shakes her head as she savors a mini chocolate cupcake. "This is a food-gasm right here," she says in awe. "Pleasure to the max for my taste buds."

Biss smiles. "If you haven't already, I want you to allow these decadent tastes and textures to ignite your senses and serve as an entrée into a realm where your sexual Pleasure exceeds the sensory extravaganza that you're having now."

"I am so down for that," Zeusse says amidst a chorus of "me too."

The screen shows video of dozens of people dancing in a sultry way on a seaside terrace at sunset—all smiling, kissing and beaming with joy. At the same time, the dancers around Biss pair off and do tango-like moves.

"My mission is to present new ideas, insights, and instructions that liberate your mind, body, and spirit from oppressive beliefs and behaviors around sexuality," Biss says, "that have kept us small, stuck, and scared, while we conform to the mold that society imposes on us from birth. This applies to all five foundations that you activate here to build your empire: Power, Pleasure, Prosperity, Protection and Peace. Each one has challenges of its own for women, but that's especially true for Pleasure."

The screen shows video of a woman walking on a beach when suddenly she stops, extends her arms to the sky and looks up with an ecstatic expression. All while purple and gold sparks explode from her body into a psychedelic swirl around her, and she closes her eyes and smiles.

"I'm here to show you," Biss says, as the dancers gyrate around her, "that Pleasure is the portal that activates your Power to create and sustain your GoddessLife. My Goddesses, repeat this with me: Pleasure is the portal that activates my Power."

You and the women say it in unison, your voices booming through the tent. At the same time, the dancers rise from their knees and shoot their arms up, facing you and the women, like human exclamation points on your statement.

"I don't get it," Andi says, gripping her coffee cup as the purple lights glimmer on her rainbow ring. "Power is public. Pleasure is private."

Biss shakes her head as the dancers kneel and lower their heads. "No, it's not. And you, Andi, are the perfect example. When you keep your sexual identity private, and therefore a secret—as you've done all your life until now—you are robbing yourself of Power to live fully and freely as who you really are in public."

"Whoah!" Andi exclaims, slamming down her coffee cup with a *clank* on the saucer. "Holy shit, man. I get it."

"And what's been holding you back?" Biss asks. "Shame, guilt and fear around your sexuality and how your family would react. Which leaves you power*less* to live and love as the true Andi."

Andi buries her face in her hands and sobs quietly.

Sunshine raises her hand. "Biss, this is like what you said, 'the personal is political,' right?"

"Exactly," Biss says. "And one of the most dramatic places that this plays out is in the bedroom. First, when you're alone, if you've been taught that it's wrong to Pleasure yourself. Second, with a male partner who wants to dictate if, when, and how you will or will not receive Pleasure. Third, if you're afraid to speak up to ask for what you want, or worse, you don't even know what you like or want because your sexuality has been so turned off."

"This makes me so fucking mad!" Marla blurts with a quavering voice. "I hate that my parents did this to me. They put me through that purity movement bullshit." Tears glisten in her eyes. "The classes, the promise ring, the brainwashing that anything sexual is a sin and that I have to wait until marriage to have sex for the purpose of having babies. The only legit thing they said was that they didn't want me to risk getting pregnant and not be

Tuesday, Day 3

able to go to college. But the way they said it was so accusatory and mean. I fucking hate them for all of it!"

Sammie joins Marla on her sofa and puts her arm around her. "I got you, Marl." Sammie pulls Marla's hair out of her face and hands her tissues.

"Marla," Biss says, "here is the place where you can heal and release that anger. I'll show you how." She looks around at all the women. "Who'd like to share if this is resonating with you?"

Sunshine raises her hand. "For me, the idea that the personal is political plays out when I'm intimate with a man who gets upset if I express what I want. Especially when I want to use my toys to make sure I orgasm like he does."

"Same!" several women exclaim.

Jade shakes her head. "That's why I like threesomes. You can enjoy the guy, and the girl will make sure you get yours."

"I'm not into that," Sunshine says. "I want my man to value my Pleasure and know that it's important for me to orgasm just like he does."

Sammie says, "I have dated so many guys who have these big, dramatic, loud orgasms, and then they're done, and look so proud about it, and don't have a clue or a care about making me cum. I freaking absolutely *hate* that, but I'm so scared to speak up when he says, 'Did you cum?' So I lie and say yes. How stupid is that!?" She looks around. "Tell me I'm not the only one who's done this."

Several women raise a hand or say "me" with a disappointed tone. Many sniffle and wipe tears.

"They get mad or insulted or give you the silent treatment," Kiki says, "if you tell the truth or ask for more. I use that as a screening process to eliminate dudes, because I don't want a real relationship. So if they're not into making sure I'm satisfied, I'm like, 'Bye, dude!'"

Delaney pipes up: "I've even faked it in my marriage, early on, just to make him feel better—"

"Porn makes guys expect a performance that is so unrealistic!" Sammie says. "But girls I know go through with all that, because there's competition. If they don't do it, someone else will. And since they want to keep the guy, and I've done this, too, they get into this role like they're some little porn star. But they're not getting off; they're just making sure the guy is happy. And sex becomes like a job."

Delaney shakes her head. "Early in our marriage, way before it was acceptable to talk about this, I got so frustrated at the unfairness, that I convinced my husband to go to a sex therapist who provided a safe, neutral space for me to express myself. Thankfully he's a wonderful, loving, caring man, and took immediate action to ensure my satisfaction. And he's been on a mission ever since to make up for all the lost orgasms."

"Beautiful," Biss says. "Later, we'll talk about closing the orgasm gap, which is like the wage gap, where women get paid less than men for the same work."

"The orgasm gap!" Kiki raises a fist in the air and looks around at the women. "Hey Biss Tribe Class number 88. Let's make it our mission to close the orgasm gap!"

Several women cheer.

Biss looks at Andi. "Andi, does this make sense now?"

"Got it," Andi says, balling her fists.

You can feel the heaviness in the air, and see the angst on many women's faces.

"Activating your GoddessPleasure," Biss says, "also activates your GoddessPower to speak up and go after everything you want in life, personally and professionally. So much so, that I believe that owning, enjoying, and even flaunting our divine right to enjoy sensual and sexual pleasure is the ultimate act of empowerment."

Tuesday, Day 3

You enjoy another bite of your dessert and sip your favorite drink as the other women nibble and listen.

"Sex is the final frontier of women's empowerment," Biss says. "Because our sexuality is taboo. For most women, it's hard to talk about, and even harder to act on, if they do at all."

Marla moans. "That's me, and my heart is like literally pounding harder with every word you say, Biss."

"Marla, you are not alone." Biss casts a comforting gaze at Marla. "And you're in the best place to find Power in your Pleasure."

The video screen fills with black and white historic images of women being punished—death by hanging in the town square or by being burned at the stake, whippings, imprisonment, and condemnation by male authority figures and villagers looking angry and pointing fingers.

"Since the beginning of time," Biss says, "women's Pleasure and Power have been stolen by oppressive cultures, religions and traditions that have used fear, guilt, shame, and even violence to confine us to patriarchal society's definition of what a woman should be."

"Sadly," she says, "some cultures mutilate female babies and girls by slicing off the clitoris and external female genitalia—with no painkiller and in very unsterile conditions, and even sewing up the vagina—to rob them of pleasure and sexual freedom."

Marla gasps. "Oh my God, that's horrible! I knew a girl in college whose village women did that to her in Africa."

Andi shakes her head. "I've read about the movement to stop it."

Biss looks disgusted as the music takes an eerie tone. "Female Genital Mutilation, according to beliefs by some cultures, is performed by women who believe it makes the woman pure, honorable and good wife material, because they believe that stealing her sexual Pleasure will keep her beholden to her husband, whose first act of intercourse with her rips open her sewn-up vagina, only to inflict pregnancies that repeatedly traumatize the non-stretchy scar tissue around her birth canal. Infections and fatal bleeding can result. More than 230 million women and girls in 30 countries in Africa, the Middle East and Asia have endured this horror."[1]

Several women groan as Zeusse exclaims, "This has to stop!"

Biss adds, "Fortunately, countries are enacting laws to ban it. Several women who've joined The Biss Tribe learned about this and made it their GoddessMission to help survivors of this and to work on a global scale to eradicate it with laws and campaigns that shift cultural beliefs and practices."

The music becomes ominous, and the women are silent as Biss continues:

"That is the extreme reality of a patriarchal society's suppression and brutal theft of women's sexuality. The rules were written by men who don't want us to discover our sexual power that is literally the birthplace of humanity. Without the female body, babies would not be born and humans would no longer exist."

Biss paces, looking angry. "This is misogyny—the hatred of women, which is all about controlling us and making us powerless. It also exists in the form of abuse, rape and murder. I believe that our Power is so extraordinary that it terrifies the patriarchy, which is socialized to control, dominate and allegedly protect. Any woman who defies those boundaries is an affront to the patriarchy, and therefore subject to punishment."

"Honor killings" appears on the screen.

"In some countries," Biss says, "male-dominated culture exerts so much power and control over women, that women can be killed by their own families if they violate strict rules prohibiting sexual behavior. If you do an online search for 'honor killings,' you'll see pictures of girls and women who were killed because they disobeyed the rules that girls are expected to follow. Oftentimes, the girl or woman's own father or male family members killed her and were acquitted of any crimes."

Biss raises her arms toward you and the women, and the music takes an upbeat tone. "Thankfully, more women like you are stepping into our Power in—business, government, entertainment, education and everywhere—forcing outdated beliefs and practices to fade into the past. But sexism and misogyny still rage."

"Fuck that!" Marla shouts. "GoddessPower! GoddessPleasure!" She raises a fist into the air. Jade, Sammie, Zeusse, Kiki, Celeste, Delaney, and many others join her, chanting, "GoddessPower! GoddessPleasure!"

As the women's voices thunder through the tent, Biss shoots her arms up, closes her eyes, and sways while the dancers go wild around her. When the chanting subsides, Biss says, "My Goddesses! Let's do this!"

The women cheer.

On the video screen, a modern woman appears; she's wearing a form-fitting dress and turning heads as she confidently strides along a bustling downtown street.

"So here's where Pleasure is the portal to our Power," Biss says. "When a woman embraces and celebrates her birthright to enjoy her body and all the glory of her six senses, as well as every aspect of her life, she rejects society's conventions on the most intimate level, and that empowers her to create a life that sparkles—explodes!—with passion and purpose."

"Halleluiah!" Celeste exclaims. "Preach it, Biss!"

The women are quiet as the dancers slowly circle Biss.

"Every one of you is a Goddess," Biss says. "So today, follow me through the GoddessPleasure Gateway into the life that you desire and deserve, and never look back. It's time and you can do it, Goddess, because *you* have the Power!"

The music booms and the dancers glimmer and shimmer around the stage. Biss steps off, and Esmerelda comes on to say: "Ladies, let's stand and stretch!"

Live Like Life is Making Love to You

After a refreshing stretch led by Esmerelda, the Concierges clear away the brunch plates, refill the flat or sparkling water in your goblets, provide fresh pots of tea and coffee and all the accompaniments, and place pretty bowls of mints, nuts and/or chocolates on each woman's table.

"I'm feeling so skeptical," Jade says to you and the women within earshot, "that I can recreate anything close to this at home. I mean, I love it. It's fantastic. But it feels like I'm watching a Las Vegas-style show featuring a motivational speech at a far-away resort."

Bianca looks anxious. "In an opulent tent eating off a silver platter of gourmet food, drinking from a gold cup—"

Andi looks pessimistic and runs a hand through her hair. "I'm scared as shit right now, because we have to take all this back and make stuff happen. I'm 61, so it's now or never. And I refuse to go to the grave without bringing that vision from the Pyramid to life. Livin' Andi's dream in my artist studio on the beach with my wife that I have to find."

"You can do it!" Sunshine exclaims, jumping up to give Andi the GoddessGreeting.

Sexy Arabic chill music booms. Biss reappears on the stage surrounded by the shimmering dancers.

"Who wants to wake up every morning," she nearly shouts, "and feel like life is making love to you so intensely, that you have multiple life-gasms throughout the day?"

"Hell yeah, baby!" Marla jumps up and cheers. Sammie does the same as the women cheer loudly.

Tuesday, Day 3

Sammie confesses, "But I'm terrified that this will open the door to ManLand."

"You have the power to script how this will play out," Biss says. "Because today, you're going to write—or rewrite—your Pleasure Story. First, I'll share mine. Then we'll start the most luscious work you'll ever do." Biss faces you and all the women.

"We have the Power to create human beings in our bodies! Think about that miracle. It's mind-blowing!"

Biss gazes at you and scans the women's faces.

"Whether you use this energy of creation to give birth to a child or children—*or not!*—that energy is still within you, and you can channel it to create *anything.* Including your Goddess empire. You just need to harness it and use it to fuel your GoddessGenius."

The dancers move slowly around Biss.

"But we live in a world where our female sexual Power is shamed, suppressed, extinguished, mutilated, assaulted, punished, killed. We're taught a long list of rules that make us feel that our natural sexuality is bad, and that if we enjoy it or pursue it, we get called all kinds of bad names that don't exist for men. Names that can destroy a reputation, a career, a sense of self. Those who fear our Power try to crush it."

The dancers shoot up, then fall flat on the floor.

"No more!" Biss shouts. "Sexual energy is one of our superpowers! So how would you like to have orgasms that are so strong and intense that it feels like your skin is sparkling with diamonds?"

Sunshine tosses her head back. "Yes, please!"

"That's what's up!" Zeusse joins the women's cheers.

"How would you like to suck Pleasure out of the most mundane tasks, and enjoy what you love even more?" Biss asks.

"Let's do it!" Celeste shouts over the women's chorus of "yes!"

"Then let's rock this," Biss says. "Start thinking about what *you* want. If you don't know, you'll set the intention in meditation later

Welcome to The Biss Tribe

today to learn from Spirit how to create your GoddessPleasure Life. So let me first share my GoddessPleasure story." The music plays softly as she speaks:

> My story starts many years ago. I've always felt free to enjoy the sexual magic of my own body, whether with self-Pleasure or while being safe and responsible with trusted lovers.
>
> At one point, after 10 years of monogamy, I was free to enjoy luscious new experiences exactly as I desired. However, discretion was a top priority, because I was a young mom dealing with an angry ex-husband. Plus, my mother had a very high-profile job in our city, and I was building a career as an author and speaker. So, reputation mattered, even though I hated the double standard that slut-shames women who dare to live freely with our sexuality.
>
> Still, I wanted to have adventurous, sexy fun. But with each lover, even when things started off like dynamite, their passion fizzled. Maybe I just wore them out! At the same time, I hated that my lovers played like I was the only one, when evidence let me know that wasn't the case. I didn't care, because I did not want a boyfriend or a husband. I just wanted to have fun.
>
> By the way, I was the queen of safe sex, demanding to see a new HIV test and insisting that they wore condoms.
>
> So why couldn't people be honest that they wanted more than one lover, and why did the thrill eventually chill?

Tuesday, Day 3

While pondering these questions, I noticed that when I paid for something—like an oil change, a teeth-cleaning or a restaurant meal—I received excellent service. So I wondered, *What if I could pay for someone to provide excellent sex for me? They could provide the service and just leave.* Well, that was illegal where I lived, so I wrote it into reality instead.

I wrote a trilogy of novels about the erotic empire of *Husbands, Incorporated.* My imagination created a fictitious company that provides fantasy marriages for women—with sexual satisfaction guaranteed by men who are trained to satisfy in every way.

Meanwhile, I *craved* this satisfaction in my own life—not with a relationship or marriage—simply with a Dream Lover who Pleasured me in an extraordinary way. Every time. This craving became especially acute after yet another relationship started as pure fire, then suddenly went terribly cold. Believe it or not, this happened at a tropical resort that should have been the perfect setting for decadent romance and passionate love-making.

Instead, I sat alone on the beach, feeling stunned, confused and sad. So I asked the Universe to deliver my Dream Lover, who would provide fiery passion and ferocious sex featuring ridiculous stamina to give me too many orgasms to count.

Here's where I used my GoddessPleasure Vision, which I'll explain shortly.

Staring out at the vast blue ocean and sky, I envisioned a man who was muscular, healthy and discreet, sharing my non-possessive, Pleasure-seeking perspective. I saw a clear vision in my mind of our first encounter, how it would look, and how it would feel.

I also emphasized that I wanted a *lover*, not a relationship, so I could focus on being a mom and a writer. I had zero desire to have a traditional relationship, fall in love or re-marry.

Back home, my relationship ended; I prayed that he would find the perfect woman, while I expressed immense gratitude to God for our peaceful parting.

A short time later, I felt my soul calling out for the man in my vision. I asked friends for referrals to eligible people, and Dream Lover came into my life.

Our first encounter played out exactly as I had envisioned. Except the Pleasure *far exceeded* my wildest expectations! Until that moment, I'd had *great* sex with amazing lovers. But Dream Lover was in a league of his own. I actually nicknamed him "the eighth wonder of the world."

Until him, I didn't know sex could be *that good*. And I didn't know that two people's body parts could fit together so perfectly, or that one stroke could ignite nerve endings throughout my entire body in a way that created indescribable Pleasure that felt like tiny diamonds were sparkling up through every inch of my skin.

During the most intense Pleasure I'd ever experienced, I saw flashes of purple and gold with fantastical visions, while psychic messages echoed in my mind. Many times, these visions and messages came from the Egyptian Goddesses Isis and Bast;

they said that Dream Lover and I had been royalty in past lives and that we were meant to reconnect in this lifetime to learn important lessons.

The extraordinary Pleasure that I experienced with this man became my benchmark for great sex. With every lover after him, I asked myself, *Did sex with them make me feel like diamonds were sparkling on my face—and my whole body? Did the extraordinary sensations elevate me into an electrifying portal where I was gifted with supernatural visions and messages?*

Unfortunately, the answer was usually no. So Dream Lover was a blessing and a curse, because he had taken me to the mountaintop, and I would rather abstain than frolic in anybody's frustrating foothills.

By the way, this practice and philosophy can apply regardless of your lover's gender or your sexual identity.

The story of my Dream Lover was my Goddess-Pleasure Awakening, which I'll explain later.

Meanwhile, being over 40 years old and experiencing such extreme Pleasure for the first time made me want to spread the gospel.

I want every woman to feel this. By the way, in perfect alignment with my request to the Universe, my Dream Lover and I didn't ever phone each other to chit-chat, exchange holiday gifts, go on dates, or try to have a "relationship." It was perfect, and underscored the philosophies about monogamy, Pleasure and women's sexual empowerment that I wrote about in *Husbands, Incorporated*.

Welcome to The Biss Tribe

I know that this type of relationship is not what many women want. But it was exactly what *I* wanted at the time. And that's key! I didn't let society or anybody else dictate *how* or *if* I would get my Pleasure. It was my decision and my choice.

And to get it, I used the manifestation tools that I'm teaching you here in The Biss Tribe.

This unique relationship enabled me to maintain my independence and focus on being a mom, a writer, a speaker—and an independent woman. It also enlivened the daily sensual extravaganza of life—food tasted better, the air felt softer, laughter sounded more joyous, and simple Pleasures like the sun on my skin felt even more luscious. It also boosted my confidence, because I felt so free to enjoy the Pleasures of my body with him.

GoddessPleasure engages and heightens all the senses, every moment of the day and night, and living in this dimension fortifies your GoddessPower on every level to build your empire.

Now I want *you* to experience that, if you so desire, whether it's with a Dream Lover who gifts you with Pleasure on your terms, or with a life partner, or in unconventional relationships.

So here's how to manifest the perfect partner, lover or relationship(s) of your own design. Use these tools that I used to manifest my Dream Lover, which were:

1. Knowing exactly what I wanted, and creating a vivid vision of what that would look and feel like for me;

Tuesday, Day 3

2. Refusing to feel that I needed to ask anyone's permission to fulfill my sexual desires;

3. Releasing any guilt, shame or fear around wanting, pursuing and getting exactly what I desired;

4. Clearly asking the infinite power of the Universe to deliver my Dream Lover;

5. Trusting that this person would adhere to my need for discretion, safety, condom use and annual STD tests;

6. Feeling that I absolutely *deserved* to have the thrill and satisfaction of this lover *on my terms*;

7. Taking action to find him by asking friends to refer and/or introduce viable candidates; and

8. Believing with patience and knowing that this like-minded and extraordinarily skilled person would come into my life.

It happened very quickly and became my longest liaison with a man since my 10 years of monogamy while married. And this non-relationship with Dream Lover was absolute bliss while it lasted.

Now it's your turn to design a life of Pleasure that suits your unique desires. You can do that by activating your GoddessPleasure here in The Biss Tribe.

"Are you ready, my gorgeous Goddesses?" Biss asks.

The women explode in cheers.

"I need to find my Dream Lover who becomes my husband!" Sunshine shouts.

A woman in the front row named Phyllis sounds annoyed as she says: "You make it sound easy to find somebody who can do all *that*. Where do I find someone like your Dream Lover?"

Welcome to The Biss Tribe

Biss steps toward her. "You *can* find your Dream Lover. Activating your GoddessPleasure energy is like programming a giant magnet inside yourself. A magnet to attract love, money, opportunities—anything you want."

Phyllis shakes her head as Biss looks at her and says, "Believe that everything we're doing here will activate your GoddessPleasure, which strengthens that magnet inside you to tap into the currents of the universe and draw in what and whom you want."

Andi scowls. "Sounds like the law of attraction. That never works for me."

"Me either," Jade snaps.

"I used to think that," Biss says. "But it didn't work for years, because I had blocks around things that needed healing. Today we'll use the GoddessPleasure Activation Tools to heal and release your blocks and help you experience your heart's desires."

Zeusse raises her hand. "Is this just about lust and sex? That's all good, but once I get my academy up and running, I want a partner who's mine and we're really in love. Exclusive. With magic in the bedroom that steals my soul."

"Same," a 40-something woman says. "I want that with my husband. We used to have it. But 15 years in, he hardly touches me and I feel so alone."

Biss casts an intense stare at you and all the women.

"Let's resolve all of the above," Biss says, "by writing or re-writing your Pleasure Story. In your *PowerJournals*, turn to the Pleasure section. Whether you're single and seeking, or partnered up and wanting to make the sex sizzle like never before, or embarking on a whole new adventure and identity, here's your chance to script your GoddessPleasure Vision."

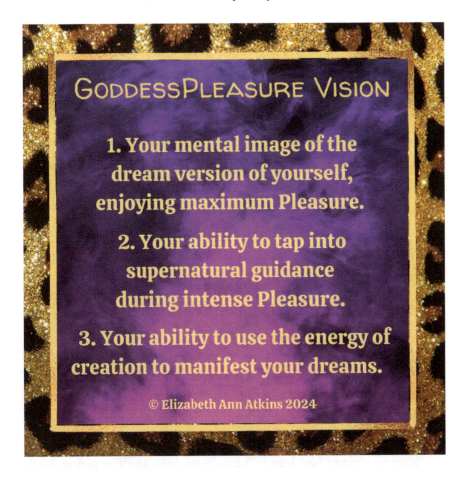

Words flash on the screen above Biss and she explains that your GoddessPleasure Vision has three parts:

1. Your mental image of the dream version of yourself, enjoying maximum Pleasure.
2. Your ability to tap into supernatural guidance during intense Pleasure.
3. Your ability to use the energy of creation to manifest your dreams.

She looks directly at you, then at each woman. "Questions?"

"That's a lot!" Bianca says.

"Will you walk us through it?" Marla asks.

"Of course," Biss says. "Today. Let's start by envisioning the types of sexual experiences that you want to make real and regular in your new life. The sky is the limit. If you want a traditional hetero-monogamous marriage, write about that. If you want to create a polyamorous 'family' of a dozen people living in a commune-type setting, write that. If you want to come out as bisexual or lesbian or another identity of your choosing, describe that. If you want to open your relationship or marriage to swing with other couples or find a unicorn playmate for threesomes, write that. If you want to be celibate, that's fine, too."

Setting GoddessPleasure Intentions in The Biss Tribe Class #88

The music softens and Biss says, "I'd like to hear each of your intentions for your GoddessPleasure. At SeaGoddess Castle, you shared what you want to accomplish by coming here. Now we're going to do that by specifically focusing on Pleasure."

Sammie raises her hand. "I kinda of feel like I'm going backwards on this, because I'm supposed to give up men for a year so I can cleanse my energy and my mind and reprogram myself, and find my perfect husband."

Biss nods. "That's what Spirit told you in the Meditarium yesterday. That does not mean that you'll abandon Pleasure. At all! In fact, the Pleasure you once sought from men, you said, had become quite miserable. So Sammie, tell us how you want to enjoy Pleasure on a daily basis as you follow the guidance to empower yourself."

Sammie's eyes widen and she shakes her head. "I am literally drawing a blank. When I think of Pleasure, I think of sex with men."

Tuesday, Day 3

Marla nudges her. "You like toys, bitch. You're even happier to play with yourself than some pump-and-squirt guy who doesn't give two shits if you cum or not."

Tears fill Sammie's eyes. "I need to rely on myself for Pleasure when it comes to sex. So, okay, I'll buy more toys! And I want to do all the things that make my body feel good, like get a massage and facials every week."

"That's a good start," Biss says. "How about you, Bianca?"

"I'll go to the symphony more," she says. "I've pushed pause on dating for now. Opening my girls' center is my top priority and I don't want to share my energy with anyone. Although I do have a lover I can call occasionally if I want, no strings attached. Pleasure? I'm going to re-read all the books about Frida Kahlo that I have in my condo, and every day I'm going to sit and look at all the beautiful artwork on my walls, and look out at San Diego Bay from my balcony while I drink my coffee and eat my favorite meals on my best China. With roses on the table. Every night!"

"That's what's up," Zeusse says, smiling.

"I want more adventure with my husband," Celeste says. "He always aims to please—halleluiah!—but our routine is so damn boring. Or we're just too tired. I want us to take romantic weekend trips. I'm going to buy more lingerie. And I want to take our couple-friends's invitation to go to a swinger's party, just to watch! I want to expand our horizons and explore exciting possibilities."

Andi raises her hand. "Man, I'm stressin' out on this one. As much as I've fantasized about it my whole life, I've never had sex with a woman. I need to find someone who can show me the ropes, so when I meet my wife, I won't be a fumbling fool about it." She runs her hand through her hair. "While I'm on the hunt for my wife, I want to date women and have sex to learn and practice."

Sunshine raises her hand. "I decided that I want to save myself for my husband. I can't believe I'm saying that, because in the past

I always thought that was naïve. You have to experience the good and the bad to know what you like and don't like. I've had enough of what I don't like. So I want to feel free to Pleasure myself and really enjoy it with no shame or guilt. I also want to enjoy more cultural celebrations. Especially Pow Wows. Nani used to take me as a girl, and I remember the joy and the spiritual energy was so strong, my whole body would have goosebumps and I'd be so happy, I'd start crying. I want to feel that again. And take time to pamper myself every day. With bubble baths, candlelight and a glass of wine."

Kiki raises her hand. "Mine is different. I want to have sex with as many people as I want. I just want to have fun with it. Safely. But I love hooking up with guys. It's exciting. I'm not scared to ask for what I want and get it. I meet guys who are excited to do whatever I ask. I don't want to be monogamous. Yuck! That bores me. I don't want a relationship and I don't know if I ever want to marry or have kids and all that. I just want to enjoy people in wild settings."

She flashes a sly smile. "Well actually that's what I already do. I just don't want to have to feel shame about it, or that I'm sneaking around, afraid my parents and brother will find out and kill me. Not literally. But they'd be really mad and tell me I dishonor the family."

Delaney waves at Biss. "It would bring me great Pleasure just by knowing that I am enough for myself and for my husband. I want to look in the mirror and love how I look at age 75. I want release the fear that I've had my entire marriage that I'm not pretty or sexy enough and that surely my husband would take a mistress who was prettier or sexier. Pleasure for me will be loving myself just as I am, knowing that I am enough in every way."

"Girlfriend," Celeste says, "I'm gonna call you every day when we leave here, and tell you that as a reminder, in case you have any off days."

Delaney smiles.

Tuesday, Day 3

"And all of us, for that matter," Celeste says. "Not enoughness is an epidemic, and it stops with all of us, right here and now."

Write Your GoddessPleasure Script

A movie theatre marquis appears on the screen and says: "Now showing: GoddessPleasure Starring YOU!"

Biss glances up at the screen and says, "We're going to script your GoddessPleasure Vision, just like we did for your Power. You're the screenwriter, creating scenes for your life. And writing is the first step to manifesting your vision in 3D reality."

The screen says "Your GoddessPleasure Script" and shows a worksheet:

Title: _____

Writer: _____

Executive Producer + Director: _____

Starring Role: _____

Heroine: _____

Hero: _____

Supporting Cast: _____

_____

Plot: _____

_____

Setting: _____

Welcome to The Biss Tribe

External Villains: _____

_____

Internal Villains: _____

_____

Ending: _____

_____

One-sentence overview:

_____

_____

Dear Goddess Reader: please complete the GoddessPleasure Script worksheet. You may want to keep reading and come back to it after you see how Biss and the 22 women complete theirs.

Biss looks at you and the women and says, "Turn to this worksheet in your *PowerJournal*. But first, let's do the exercise together. Who wants to volunteer as our example?"

Marla's hand shoots up. "I do!" She glances around as if to ask permission from the women.

"Go for it!" Sunshine says enthusiastically.

"Do your thing," Zeusse adds.

Biss nods. "Yes, Marla."

Tuesday, Day 3

Marla grimaces. "Like I said at SeaGoddess Castle, I'm royally fucked up about sex, because my super Christian parents made me do purity culture and our Filipino community in LA—I love them—but my dad is a pastor and under his influence, they all made me cray-cray about it. So much, that I've never had an orgasm. Never had sex with a guy. Too scared. Total impostor syndrome as an influencer whose brand is super sexy."

"Good summary," Biss says. "Now tell me the title of your GoddessPleasure script."

"Free, Freaky and Authentically Me," Marla says as Esmerelda types on a laptop and her answers appear on the screen above the stage.

"Yes, bitch!" Sammie shrieks.

"Excellent!" Biss beams. The music blasts. And the dancers explode in a frenzy. "Marla, you're the writer, executive producer, director and heroine. So who's your supporting cast? Include me, Esmerelda, and your 21 Biss Tribe sisters who bring our talent and support to the table. Who else?"

"Sammie," Marla says. "She's my supporting actress. I feel like liberating myself will launch our skincare line, Samla-Marmie, in a whole new way."

Biss nods. "Who's the hero?"

"I want to experience different men before I get married," Marla says. "So I kinda need a cast of men as a sort of screening or interview process for my husband. So the ultimate hero is the man I marry."

"Plot?" Biss asks.

"A sexually oppressed influencer and entrepreneur suffering from imposter syndrome unlocks her mind and body from religious-guilt prison after being put there by her family's religious shaming. She finds her power in her Pleasure, becomes multi-orgasmic, has safe and great sex with men, and finds a husband who loves her inner freak, and all that makes her the most bad ass girl boss ever."

"You nailed it!" Sammie shouts as several women cheer and clap.

"Setting?" Biss asks.

"Miami where I live, but also LA where my parents are," Marla says, "and really the world, because we travel so much."

Biss nods. "Who are your external villains?"

"My parents, my extended family and the church community," Marla says. "Online trolls who are sex-shamers. And really society, because there's so much messaging that tries to make us feel bad about being sexy."

"Internal villains?" Biss asks.

"It's me!" Marla says sadly. "It's the fucked-up programming inside my head that has shut down my body. Like—" she looks around nervously. "Remember the confidentiality here, bitches."

"You're safe," Biss says. "What's said in the Pleasure Tent stays in the Pleasure Tent. Everybody in agreement? Say yes."

You and the women say yes, and Marla says, "If I touch myself, it's like my whole brain goes crazy and I can literally hear all the garbage they said to me, like, *Whores suffer in hell and burn forever in a lake of fire.* That is so caveman era!"

Marla wipes tears from her eyes. "Even though my parents disowned me and I hate them for making me this way, I want to live my life for me and reunite with my family in a way that they accept and love me."

Biss casts a sympathetic look at Marla. "You can make that happen. Now, can you give us a one-sentence summary?"

"GoddessPleasure makes Marla Santos sexually free and happy, super successful in business, and reunited with her loving family."

Several women clap.

"It's hard to fit all that in one sentence," Andi says. "Good job!"

Tuesday, Day 3

"I am like shaking inside to do this," Jade says. "For me, music is pure Pleasure. Writing, listening, performing and doing everything around it. I'm not really inhibited with men or women, or myself. But I have to shake this sad feeling that I'm alone right now, even though deep down, I know that's best for me to figure things out."

Sunshine looks around nervously. "Same! Sometimes my body has wanted self-Pleasure, but after I do it, I burst into tears because I want so bad to have a man who can share that with me. It's a reminder that I'm alone and that I haven't found my husband yet."

Biss casts a comforting stare at Jade and Sunshine. "So now's your time to script exactly what you want. Just like we did at SeaGoddess Castle, let it play out like a movie in your imagination until your GoddessPleasure becomes your daily reality. Be delusional and unrealistic!"

She holds up a *PowerJournal*. "Open your book to the page that says: **My GoddessPleasure Vision.** We're going to write the vision from your conscious imagination, which is your thinking mind, right now. Then we'll meditate later and fill in more details and action steps."

Celeste asks, "Biss, do we have to do this exercise with a partner or solo?"

"Today, you can do it privately by writing," Biss says as the music becomes mellow. "Now in your mind, ask your Supernatural Self to help you write your GoddessPleasure Vision. Ask her to quiet the noise in your head, so you can focus on writing the most luscious vision for your life. Then ask your Supernatural Self to upload the images into an imaginary projector that makes your vision play like a film on your mental movie screen."

Welcome to The Biss Tribe

Dear Goddess Reader:

Write a detailed scene from your GoddessPleasure Life and/or use the audio recording app on your phone to describe it verbally. Then read and/or listen to your description every morning and night.

_____

_____

_____

_____

After 20 minutes of writing, a loud chime sounds and Biss asks, "How was that?"

"For me," Zeusse says, "it's clear. I know what I want. A boo who's as busy and ambitious as myself, so we can hook up when we can, but I stay free to build my girls basketball academies, while she does her thing."

"What about your Pleasure?" Biss asks.

"I got some stuff to work on," Zeusse says. "So I wrote some ways to have Pleasure every day by myself. Like, this might sound crazy, but I love to go to this bath house in Harlem and just sit in the steam and chill. The heat, the sweat, the zenned-out feeling, that's my happy place. But I haven't gone in a long time. Now I'ma go at least once a week."

"Nice," Andi says.

"What about sexual Pleasure?" Biss asks.

"I want to find my boo who's got the perfect chemistry with me. The whole thing. Mind, body, soul. In perfect synch. Like you said, the new standard, with no hang-ups. I also need to meditate on cleaning out stuff that Mama G said that still lingers in my head."

Biss nods. "We'll be doing a healing meditation for that."

"That's what's up," Zeusse says.

Tuesday, Day 3

Find Your Pleasure by Identifying How You Feel Pleasureless

The screen shows a diagram as Biss says, "Please look at this diagram in your *PowerJournal*."

With MYSELF	How do I feel pleasureless?	What would make me feel Pleasure?	How to find my Pleasure.
With Other People & in the World	How do I feel pleasureless?	What would make me feel Pleasure?	How to find my Pleasure.
With Spirit	How do I feel pleasureless?	What would make me feel Pleasure?	How to find my Pleasure.

"Let's look at how you feel pleasureless," Biss says, "so you can know where you need to boost your Pleasure the most."

Delaney raises a hand. "What do you mean by pleasureless with Spirit?"

"If you feel that the only messaging and guidance you get from Spirit is bad," Biss says. "Shaming you, condemning you, telling you what you *can't* be or do. That God is mad at you for having impure thoughts."

Jade asks, "Does that mean it's not coming from Spirit and it's actually from our own heads?"

"Yes, it's coming from deeply-ingrained societal programming. So we'll work on reprogramming our minds and creating a clear channel to Spirit so we can hear our GoddessVoice speak the truth, which is all about enabling you to enjoy Pleasure as long as it's not harming you or anyone else."

"I love that," Sunshine says.

"So let's take five minutes to fill in this worksheet," Biss says. "Leave the 'how to' column blank. We're going to meditate later to get your action steps."

After five minutes, the chime sounds. Suddenly a male dancer and a female dancer swing through the air above the stage. They're on gold boards held by ropes and suspended from a horizontal pole across the ceiling that's fortified by vertical poles.

"Oh my Goddess!" Marla gushes as dramatic music booms.

"Holy shit!" Andi says.

Several women gasp in surprise, and all are mesmerized by the *Cirque du Soleil*-type performance as the dancers—wearing skimpy, bejeweled costumes—defy gravity with graceful moves on the swings. A gold circle drops and dangles between them, and the dancers slip onto it, twisting and twirling like poetry in motion, gazing at each other with love and teasing their bodies together with sensuous movements.

Zeusse watches in awe. "Life-gasm, for sure."

Tuesday, Day 3

Your GoddessPleasure Awakening

A definition for GoddessPleasure Awakening appears on the screen.

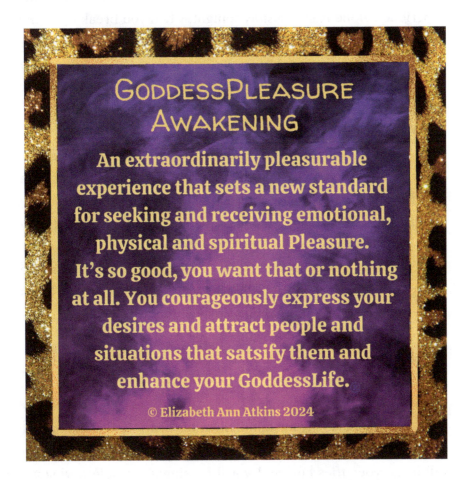

"During my Dream Lover story," Biss says, "I said that experience was my GoddessPleasure Awakening, which is an extraordinarily pleasurable experience that sets a new standard for seeking and receiving emotional, physical and spiritual Pleasure. It's so good, you want that or nothing at all. It makes you courageously express your desires and attract people and situations that satisfy them and enhance your GoddessLife."

Sunshine raises her hand. "How do we know if we've had that awakening yet?"

"Oh, you'll know!" Biss smiles. "Because it will blow your mind. It will be unprecedented and unparalleled. You may have this experience alone first. Possibly tonight, when you break open the toybox in your private tent and start exploring your own erogenous zones."

"OhmyGod," Marla says. "I'm so embarrassed right now; my cheeks feel hot."

"Me too," several women echo.

Zeusse raises her hand. "I had my awakening with my first experience. I was only 16, and this older female in my building, she was like 30 at the time, she showed me how it's supposed to be."

Kiki adds, "That happened with me and an older guy. I'd only been with guys my age, and this guy had me on a whole nother level. At first it was so intense, it freaked me out, because he brought out dildos and this vibrator that you plug in and it looks like a microphone. A Doxy wand. He used that with a dildo on me—with a vibrating butt plug—"

"Holy shit," Andi says playfully, "my virgin ears!"

Kiki laughs. "And I swear that orgasm was like 10 minutes long. I slept for 12 hours after that."

Celeste smiles. "My husband, bless his heart, is also hip to that program. Or we use the wand during intercourse. Girlfriend, *that* will make your toes curl and you'll be singin' a whole new song. Literally."

Biss raises her arms in praise. "Yes! Thank you for sharing."

"I want to feel that," Andi says.

"Me too," Sunshine adds.

The music booms, the dancers spin around Biss, and she says, "Then let's talk about how you can step through your GoddessPleasure Gateway."

Tuesday, Day 3

Let's Step Through the GoddessPleasure Gateway

A golden gateway appears on the screen above Biss.

"Remember the Gateway exercise? Well now we're going to step through the GoddessPleasure Gateway. A long list of things may be blocking you from enjoying the vision of your GoddessPleasure Life that you just wrote about. So now's our chance to identify what those blocks are, and learn the action steps to blast past them into your most decadent existence."

Words pop onto the screen and Biss reads:

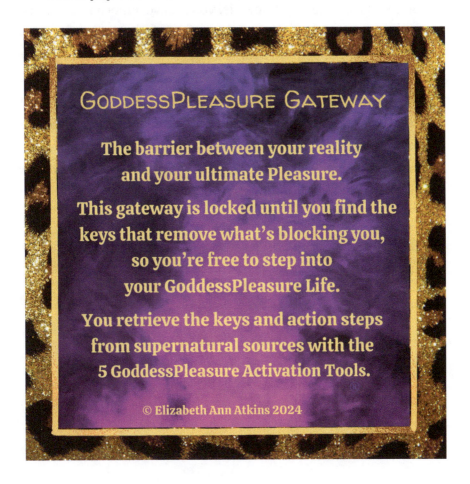

"Your GoddessPleasure Gateway is the barrier between your reality and your ultimate Pleasure. This gateway is locked until you find the keys that remove what's blocking you, so you're free to step into your GoddessPleasure Life. You retrieve the keys and action steps from supernatural sources by using the five GoddessPleasure Activation Tools."

The dancers step in front of her, forming a human wall. Then they part and she steps through. "Who's ready to step through the Gateway?"

The women cheer.

"I need a tornado to come and rip open my gate," Marla says.

Biss smiles. "The good news is, you'll have supernatural assistance to do this. Just like in the Meditarium. So no matter how much cement, barbed wire or thorny vines are blocking your gateway, it's no match for the Power of Spirit."

Biss points up at the diagram on the screen. "Let's look at where you are now and where you want to be in terms of Pleasure. You may relate to some of the issues under the Current Reality column and you may want to experience some of the things under the GoddessPleasure column. Any thoughts?"

Tuesday, Day 3

Step through the GoddessPleasure Gateway to your happiest you!

Current Reality
- lack of pleasure + feeling unsatisfied
- guilt, shame, fear around self-pleasure
- discomfort with body image
- not feeling worthy of pleasure
- wanting a lover to legitimize pleasure
- needing permission to indulge
- self-punishment / self-sabotage
- health issues that hinder pleasure
- thinking that pleasure is limited to sex
- not knowing what you like or want
- fearing risks

GoddessPleasure
- enjoying pleasure
- bliss + better moods
- feeling satisfied
- safe & secure
- confident & worthy!
- wellness benefits
- attracting loving relationships
- learning what you like
- integrating pleasure into every aspect of daily life

Action Steps
- Action Step 1
- Action Step 2
- Action Step 3
- Action Step 4
- Action Step 5
- Action Step 6
- Action Step 7
- Action Step 8
- Action Step 9
- Action Step 10
- Action Step 11
- Action Step 12

© Elizabeth Ann Atkins 2024

The Bliss Tribe Retreat

Delaney raises her hand. "I know a lot of women who hit menopause and everything changes. They lose sexual desire. They dry out and have pain during sex. They gain weight and don't feel good about themselves. They're more worried than ever that their husbands will cheat with a younger woman. Etcetera."

Biss nods. "Please, Delaney, when you go home, tell them to join The Biss Tribe to help them gracefully ease into that next season of life with the Power and Pleasure that they deserve. Please."

Delaney nods.

"That's for all of you," Biss says. "You're getting solid solutions here, and when people see you glow up into the Goddess that you are, personally and professionally, they'll want to know how you did it. Tell them. The more empowered women we have in the world, the better the world will be."

"Amen!" Celeste exclaims as several women say "Yes!" and cheer.

"So now," Biss says, pointing up at the next diagram on the screen, "let's take five minutes to fill out this worksheet to show where you are now and where you want to be in terms of Pleasure. Remember to leave the third column blank. We'll get the action steps during meditation this afternoon."

Tuesday, Day 3

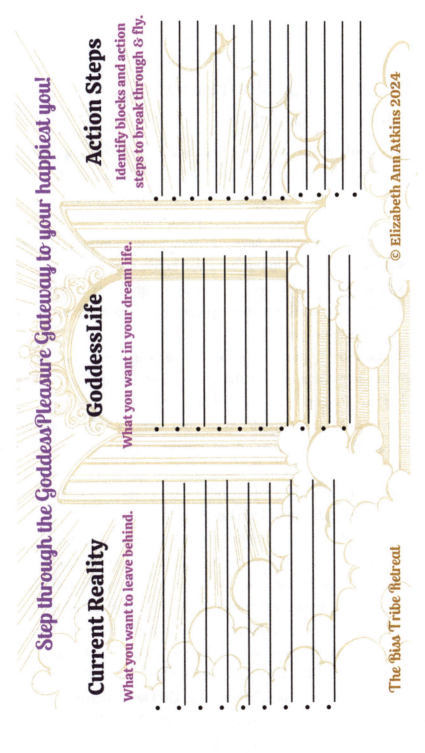

Step through the GoddessPleasure Gateway to your happiest you!

Action Steps
Identify blocks and action steps to break through & fly.

GoddessLife
What you want in your dream life.

Current Reality
What you want to leave behind.

The Bliss Tribe Retreat

© Elizabeth Ann Atkins 2024

After five minutes, chimes sound and Biss says, "Let's take a break to boost our energy! Everybody, come down to the stage!"

Activate Your GoddessPleasure with Sensuous Movement

As you and the women join Biss and Esmerelda on the stage, beautiful music plays; it's a global fusion of chimes, drumming, guitars and a female vocalist hitting satiny notes without words. A Concierge brings Bianca and her powerchair.

"Ladies," Esmerelda says, "a tremendous amount of energy gets stored and stuck in our hips and pelvis area. This energy can be shame and limiting beliefs about our sensuality and sexuality. We need to release this stored-up energy in order to truly activate our GoddessPleasure."

Esmerelda begins to move her hips in wide, slow circles. "Sensuous movement and dance can help awaken that energy and get it circulating through your body. So feel the music pulsing through you, and gently sway your hips with the intention of releasing that powerful Kundalini energy in and around your root chakra and sacral chakra."

You and the women mimic her movements.

"This reminds me of hula hooping," Kiki says.

Esmerelda raises her hands toward the ceiling and says, "Raise your arms over your head and let them sway like antennas connecting to divine energy that can help release any emotions, experiences and traumas that may be stored in our feminine energy bodies. Allow the gentle dance movements to loosen your muscles and your energetic grip on anything we need to heal and release."

"This is nice," Delaney says, closing her eyes and dancing.

Esmerelda continues: "Allow your GoddessVoice to guide your movement. She'll tell you how to move intuitively."

You and the women become one gentle flow of arms, legs and peaceful faces.

"Spin if you want," Esmerelda says. "Let the Spirit move you. Shift your weight from one foot and hip to the other, back and forth."

Then she demonstrates as she speaks: "Raise one shoulder and move it back, guiding your hip to do the same. Then do that with your other shoulder and hip."

Andi struggles to follow along, but grins. "Man, I love this."

"You can do it anytime at home," Esmerelda says. "Simply play sensuous music with the intention of activating the sexual Pleasure centers in your body."

"Very zen," says Zeusse, who's taller than everyone and swaying in the center of the women.

Soon the performers from earlier join all of you on the stage, the music takes on a faster beat, and everyone is dancing.

"A pop-up dance party!" Sunshine says. "I am blissing out on this."

Let's Talk about Sacred Sexuality

After the energizing dance and bathroom break, you and the women return to your sofas, where the Concierges refill your beverages.

At the same time, the dancers help Esmerelda set up her Tibetan sound bowls and her drum in a semi-circle on a plush blanket on the stage. She strikes a tone on a bowl and begins her wordless song that sounds like silk streaming through the air.

"Let's talk about sacred sexuality," Biss says, standing on the stage. "Sacred means connected with God/Spirit/Universe. Sexuality relates to our feelings, thoughts, identities and behaviors that stimulate Pleasure in our erogenous zones. Sacred sexuality merges our spirituality with our physical senses."

The women are silent and still, listening with rapt attention.

"In terms of GoddessPower and GoddessPleasure," Biss says, "sacred sexuality is one of our superpowers. It is the fusion of your Supernatural Self and your physical senses in a way that opens spiritual channels to heal you, provide divine guidance and elevate your mind, body and soul. You can experience this by yourself. And if you choose to have a soul mate partner, you can seize the power of this experience together."

The screen shows video of two people whose bodies are united as colorful energy explodes around them.

"Sacred sexuality is the most magical and mystical experience that we can have," Biss says, "and once we master it, we can have full-body orgasms along with psychedelic experiences that provide visions and divine messages that accompany intense and indescribable physical pleasure. Again, it can happen whether you're alone or with a partner. I've experienced both, and I want that for you, too."

The screen above Biss shows the words "spiritual" and "sexual." She looks at you and all the women. "Who has a hard time with these two words together?"

A chorus of "Me!" thunders through the tent.

"It's like the ultimate contradiction," Marla says.

"Polar opposites," Andi adds.

"One is dirty, one is clean," Sammie says. "Like, you can't be both."

"Yes!" Biss exclaims, standing up. "Yes you can! First, let's talk about religion versus spirituality. A lot of people who've been wounded by religion, especially around sexuality, reject it—"

"As in, me, Marla Santos!"

Biss nods. "As a result, millions of people now ascribe to the idea of being 'spiritual, not religious.' While religion follows a certain rulebook, such as the Christian Bible or the Jewish Torah,

Tuesday, Day 3

spirituality includes all of the Divine and allows you to define your own beliefs and create your own practices."

The screen shows video of angels and divine beings amidst pastel clouds and sunbeams.

"And while religion often shames and condemns sexuality, causing lifetime traumas," Biss says, "spirituality is all-loving and liberating. It doesn't require other humans—usually men—to define and enforce its rules. It frees you to do that for yourself."

"One hundred percent!" Zeusse nods. "That's what's up."

"Unfortunately, society's rules around women's sexuality are rooted in religious doctrine," Biss says, "and those rules are taught and enforced by families and society. It's time to reject those rules!"

Biss shoots her arms in the air and declares: "We can be deeply spiritual and highly sexual at the same time!"

Images of the Virgin Mary and a prostitute appear on the screen.

"I totally reject the virgin-whore syndrome that society has promulgated from the beginning of time," Biss says. "This phenomenon—that a woman is either a pure virgin *or* a dirty whore—is presented in most religious teachings. This is also called the Madonna-whore syndrome, which categorizes women on the two extremes of being praised as virginal and pure like Mother Mary, or scorned for being sexually promiscuous."

Many women shout, "Boo!"

"We're all somewhere in between," Jade declares. "There should be no shame, even for people who choose to be sex workers."

Biss shakes her head. "I could rant for five hours about this. If you want to dive deeper into this topic, you can read *Healing Religious Hurts: Stories & Tips to Find Love and Peace*, a book that I co-authored with former Catholic nun Joanie Lindenmeyer, who married a woman and proudly proclaims her love for Jesus and God."

Welcome to The Biss Tribe

The purple book cover appears on the screen as Biss paces the stage. "Most religious doctrine was written by men and is enforced by men. Their rules laid the foundation for society's oppressive playbook for how women should live and love."

The image of a sexy, buff man appears on the screen. "We all know that a promiscuous man is praised as a stud, a lady's man, or a Casanova. And even if they commit adultery or break the law, they often go unpunished."

The words "slut shaming" appear on the screen. "On the contrary," Biss says, "slut-shaming is society's tool for punishing women who are sexually liberated, and social media and AI make it easier than ever to hurt girls and women. It can be so traumatic that some choose suicide."

Sounds of disgust erupt throughout the tent.

"The bottom line for us here today is that this unfairness guilts and shames women," Biss says, "sometimes so profoundly that it shuts down their ability to enjoy sex or even orgasm. We're here to change that by activating our GoddessPleasure. And like our GoddessPower, it's activated by supernatural sources."

Biss raises her index finger. "But first, let's resolve the false perception that a woman cannot be deeply spiritual and highly sexual at the same time. During my year-long spiritual retreat, I spent every day meditating, doing yoga, eating a strict vegan plant-based diet, praying, journaling, and writing books. I ate no meat or dairy, had no sex and very little social life, only listened to gospel or spiritual music, and blocked out the noisy world. My spiritual connection was psychic and psychedelic, and I was in my GoddessGenius Zone as never before. During that time, I wrote my erotic trilogy, *Husbands, Incorporated.*"

The book cover appears on the screen, showing the silhouette of a man's buff chest.

Tuesday, Day 3

"However," Biss says, "writing erotica seemed totally incongruous with my extraordinary spiritual experiences. How could I simultaneously be a spiritual teacher talking about the power of God within us, and be an erotica writer presenting radical viewpoints about marriage and monogamy? This question made my heart pound with anxiety. So I meditated about it."

The screen shows video of Biss meditating in a lush garden. "Spirit answered that it's part of my life's mission to show the world that a woman can integrate the erotic and the spiritual. So *Husbands, Inc.* became my literary response to a global society where men typically make the rules about women's sexuality. In my books, women make the rules, flex the power, and are guaranteed Pleasure. And you get to hear Husbands, Inc. co-founder Venus Roman at the GoddessPleasure feast tonight on the terrace."

"Yes!" Celeste exclaims. "She and Raye Johnson are my sheroes."

A photo of Venus and Raye appears on the screen. Venus is tall and slim, with suntanned skin and short blond hair and she's wearing a white business skirt-suit. Raye has a mane of black hair framing her flawless, milk chocolate complexion and fiery eyes, and she's wearing a dark pinstriped pantsuit.

Biss beams up at their photo. "You'll meet Husbands, Inc. co-founder Raye Johnson tomorrow at the Treasure Cave, when she speaks about GoddessProsperity at the evening feast."

The words "sacred sexuality" reappear on the screen.

"So my Goddesses, talk to me," Biss says. "How is this resonating with you?"

"This is hard!" Bianca says. "It goes against everything I was taught."

Sunshine crosses her arms. "It makes me furious that we've been brainwashed in ways that steal our joy. I'm done with that!"

Delaney nods. "I have many friends my age who never awaken to the fact that we have the Power to define and enjoy our sexual Pleasure. I intend to share these insights with them."

Marla wipes her nose with tissues. "I want to leave here, like fully able to enjoy my own body."

"You will," Biss says. "So let's get back to the word sacred. That was my ultimate aspiration in finding my perfect mate. I asked the Universe to send me a man who wanted with me all that I wanted with him: a loving, passionate partnership that fulfills us on every level, with zero desire for other people. Not because that's how it quote 'should' be. But because we both genuinely feel that way."

Sunshine claps.

"And I wanted a profound connection on an emotional, physical and spiritual level," Biss says, "that is equally reciprocated and that evolves to ever-higher heights of bliss, comfort and fun every day."

Sunshine raises the back of her hand to her forehead and playfully swoons. "Oh my goodness! I want that so bad!"

"But is that really possible?" Jade asks. "Most men can't keep it in their pants, even when they're in love."

"It doesn't have to be a man," Zeusse says.

"Girls cheat, too," Jade says. "Gay girls and straight girls."

Biss continues: "When we activate our GoddessPleasure, it *is* possible to draw in someone who will honor you. The secret is to attune your Supernatural Self to such a high frequency, after healing and releasing whatever is blocking you, so that you become a magnet to draw that extraordinary person to you."

"Let's do that!" Sunshine says. "Now!"

Tuesday, Day 3

Using the Five GoddessPleasure Activation Tools

The screen lists the GoddessPleasure Activation Tools:

1. Pranayama breathing
2. Energy/chakra clearing
3. Meditation
4. Journaling
5. Orgasmic visualization

A murmur ripples through the tent.

"What in the world is orgasmic visualization?" Andi asks.

Biss flashes a fun smile. "Oh, you'll see. For now, let's start by using the four Activation Tools that you learned at the GoddessPower Pyramid, with a focus on activating your Pleasure."

As Esmerelda continues to play her sound bowls and sing on the stage, Biss sits nearby on a thick, round purple velvet pillow that has gold tassels on the sides.

"First," she says, "sit with your legs crossed or extended, and keep your spine straight and your chin level. Also, keep your *PowerJournals* handy to record the guidance that you're about to receive from Spirit during meditation."

You and the women follow the instructions.

"The difference between yesterday and today is our intention," Biss says. "Today we're setting the intention to focus on Pleasure. You'll be asking Spirit to show you the most grandiose version of yourself, experiencing your ultimate GoddessPleasure. You'll also ask to learn what's blocking you and how to remove those blocks and step into your dream life."

Biss presses her thumb to one nostril. "Let's start with Pranayama breathing. Press your thumb to one nostril to close it. Inhale deeply through the other side of your nose. Then press the tip of your ring finger to the other nostril, press it closed, and exhale through the opposite nostril."

You and the women follow her lead.

"Inhale so deeply that your belly pokes out slightly," Biss says, "and become aware of the sensations of that delicious, fresh air flowing into your body, followed by the old air leaving. Let's do this four times on each side."

As Biss does the breathing exercise, she says, "Breath is our life force. Infusing our brains and bodies with fresh oxygen helps us relax, rejuvenate and activate our greatest GoddessPleasure. Now let's inhale peace, and exhale anxiety. Breathe in faith... exhale fear. Inhale serenity... exhale shame. Breathe in courage... exhale guilt."

Dear Goddess Reader: You can watch a video demonstration of Pranayama on the YouTube channel for The Goddess Power Show with Elizabeth Ann Atkins® by using this QR code:

Tuesday, Day 3

After four repetitions, Biss asks, "Who has an oxygen buzz?"

"Me," Jade says with a mellow tone. "I'm gonna do this before every performance. I love it."

Biss smiles. "Now it's time to cleanse our energy bodies with a shower of light and a sound bath."

The lights dim and Esmerelda continues her soothing sound bowl music and wordless song. Biss holds up a *PowerJournal*. "Remember you'll journal about any guidance that you receive during the meditation. Turn to the page that says GoddessPleasure Vision Meditation number one."

Dear Goddess Reader: Please use this QR code to hear or watch Biss leading this energy clearing, meditation and journaling exercise.

GoddessPower Tools

Welcome to The Biss Tribe

Biss speaks in a soothing tone:

> Sit with your spine straight. Close your eyes and become very aware of your breath, your face and your body. Notice any tension in your forehead, your jaw, your neck, your back and anywhere else. Then envision those muscles as if they're butter, growing warmer and softer, melting away all tension into a warm, sweet flow circulating through your body.
>
> Now let's set the intention to clear our energy, get into a deeply relaxing state of meditation, connect with the Divine and learn the guidance we need to bring our GoddessPleasure Visions into 3-D reality. We want to ask Spirit to reveal the most grandiose vision of you enjoying your ultimate GoddessPleasure, along with what's blocking you and what action steps you need to take to step through the Gateway where Pleasure is one of the five foundations of your GoddessLife.
>
> Now imagine you're walking outside, onto the grass. As you look up at the sky, a golden beam of sparkling light shoots down to consume your entire being. This powerful pillar of light pulses all around you and through you, glowing like a crown of light above you, then pouring its warm, golden glow—like a shower of light—into your head, cascading down your throat, through your chest, your arms and out your fingertips, extending into your abdomen, then surging down your legs and shooting tiny lightning bolts from your feet into the ground.

Tuesday, Day 3

Envision this light shooting from your tailbone into the earth, through the mud, rocks and water, then anchoring to the core of Mother Earth. Now imagine that this pillar of light is surging up from the center of earth, through your body and up into the infinity of sky and space.

As this luminescent beam pulsates up and down, creating a crystalline column of light anchored in the Earth and plugging you into the infinite energy of the universe, you are the connecting point between heaven and earth, with your heart at the very center.

Now in your heart space, envision someone whom you love more than anyone. Savor that feeling of pure love and joy. See the light shower pouring through you and illuminating that love, expanding it outward from your heart, filling your entire body, then bursting into a joyous bubble around you.

Imagine this love brightening the light inside your body, illuminating every cell. See this light that's infused with love going into every cell in your body like tiny sparkles, burning away any bacteria, toxins, viruses or mutations. See that light and love restoring every cell in your body to perfect health and repairing your DNA to perfection. Again, see this love and light shooting like laser beams into your cells to deactivate and destroy any toxins, bacteria, viruses and mutations, restoring every cell to immaculate health.

Imagine this sparkling bright light from heaven pulsing through your veins and arteries, purifying your blood, your muscles and your bones. See it surging up into your brain, where it makes your synapses fire with perfect precision, restoring and maintaining optimum chemical balance for your mental health, and enabling all your body functions to operate in perfect synchronicity.

See the love and light illuminating your brain's left lobe, right lobe, pineal gland, prefrontal cortex, reticular activating system, subconscious mind, brain stem and your spinal cord.

Now this light infused with love expands through your skull, your scalp, into your hair, then into your eyes and ears to protect your vision and hearing. Next, this cleansing light flows into your respiratory system to infuse your nose, mouth, throat and lungs with supernatural immunity. Yes, your respiratory system is filled with this beautiful and powerful light, making you immune to any bacteria, toxins, viruses or mutations.

Next, this light cascades into your heart, where it heals both heartache and physical ailments. See this light flowing into your stomach, pancreas, gallbladder, spleen, liver, kidneys, intestines and reproductive organs.

Witness how this light floods your nervous system, your adrenal glands, your lymph nodes, even your fat, before it expands outward to restore your skin to perfect health.

See this light glowing around you, then circling the entire world with peace and love to bless every person with nourishment, safety, shelter, education, clean air, clean water, freedom of speech, freedom of religion and all good things.

Tuesday, Day 3

See this light making the leaders of the countries doing good things for the people and the planet, while Mother Earth is restored to her majestic glory. Then see the light swirling back to your home country, blessing every person with peace and love, safety, equality and justice. Then see this light surrounding your loved ones like tiny tornadoes of light that infuse them with supernatural immunity while creating a forcefield of supernatural protection around each one. See their faces glowing with health and happiness.

Now see all that light pouring into the top of your head like a shower of golden sparks, cascading through you, and washing over the energy field around and within your body. Feel this light clearing away negative energy and opening the channels to connect to the universal field of knowledge and the Divine, while boosting your immunity and cultivating wellness in mind, body and spirit.

See this light pooling at your tailbone, swirling around your ruby red **Root Chakra**. Spirit, please cleanse and clear our Root Chakras, to empower our ability to survive and thrive with courage and success in physical, sexual and financial health, which all enhance and intensify our GoddessPleasure. The tone is *Lam*. Inhale and say it with me. The tone will create a vibration that is a sound bath that clears the energy of your Root Chakra. Imagine that this sound bath is removing any smudges, smog or dimness around your ruby red Root Chakra, while making it spin and circulate its powerful energy through your entire being.

Biss, you and all the women inhale and join a long, loud, extended chant of: "Laaaaaaaaaaahhhmmmmmm." The vibration is loud and powerful in your ears as it reverberates through your body.

"Above our now glowing and spinning ruby red Root Chakra and below the navel is the orange **Sacral Chakra**," Biss says. "It represents creativity and sensuality. Spirit, please cleanse and clear our Sacral Chakras, so that we may enjoy emotional balance, creativity, sensual bliss and our infinite GoddessPleasure. The tone is *Vam*. Inhale and say it with me. Imagine that this sound bath is removing any smudges, smog or dimness around your orange Sacral Chakra, while making it spin and circulate its powerful energy through your entire being."

Biss, you, and all the women inhale and join a long, loud, extended chant of: "Vaaaaaaaaaaahhhmmmmmm."

"Next," Biss says, "our yellow **Solar Plexus Chakra** above the navel rules personal power and action. Spirit, please cleanse and clear our Solar Plexus Chakras, to empower us to confidently and courageously take aggressive action to enjoy GoddessPleasure every day. The tone is *Ram*. Inhale and chant it with me. Imagine that this sound bath is removing any smudges, smog or dimness around your yellow Solar Plexus Chakra, while making it spin and circulate its powerful energy through your entire being."

The Meditarium vibrates with you, Biss and the women chanting in unison: "Raaaaaaaaaaahhhhmmmmm."

"Next is the emerald-green **Heart Chakra** at the center of your chest, and it rules unconditional love and healing," Biss says. "Spirit, please cleanse and clear our Heart Chakras, so that we can give and receive unconditional love and healing, and enjoy GoddessPleasure in romance and love, free of inhibitions and unhindered by hurts of the past. The tone is *Yam*. Inhale and say it together. Imagine that this sound bath is removing any smudges, smog or dimness around your emerald-green Heart Chakra, while making it spin and circulate its powerful energy through your entire being."

"Yaaaaaaaaaahhhmmmmmm," everyone chants.

"Above that is the turquoise **Throat Chakra**, which rules communication," Biss says. "Spirit, please cleanse and clear our Throat Chakras, to empower our ability to express our highest truths with courage and confidence, to demand honesty from others, and to express our wildest desires to experience our ultimate GoddessPleasure. The tone is *Ham*; inhale and chant together. Imagine that this sound bath is removing any smudges, smog or dimness around your turquoise Throat Chakra, while making it spin and circulate its powerful energy through your entire being."

"Haaaaaaaaaahhhmmmmmm," echoes through the Meditarium.

"Next, your indigo **Third Eye Chakra** between the eyebrows rules intuition," Biss says. "Spirit, please cleanse and clear our Third Eye Chakras, to empower our ability to see into the divine realm and get a clear view of our GoddessPleasure Vision, along with guidance on how to remove obstacles and manifest our wildest desires, as we build our personal and professional empires. The tone is *Sham*. Inhale and say it together. Imagine that this sound bath is removing any smudges, smog or dimness around your indigo Third Eye Chakra, while making it spin and circulate its powerful energy through your entire being."

Everyone chants: "Shaaaaaaaaaahhhmmmmmm."

"Now, at the top of your head is the lavender **Crown Chakra**, which represents divine connection," Biss says. "Spirit, please cleanse and clear our Crown Chakras, to empower our spiritual awakening, self-realization and unity with Source, humanity and all divine guidance to bring our GoddessPleasure Visions to life. The tone is *Om*. Inhale and let's chant together, three times. Imagine that this sound bath is removing any smudges, smog or dimness around your lavender Crown Chakra, while making it spin and circulate its powerful energy through your entire being.""

"Ooooooooooooohhhmmmmmm."

"Ooooooooooooohhhmmmmmm."

"Ooooooooooooohhhmmmmmm."

The room is silent as Biss says: "Now that you're in a very relaxed state, I'm going to guide you on a meditation to connect with Spirit and learn more about your GoddessPleasure Vision, as well as the action steps you need to take to enter the gateway and make extraordinary Pleasure part of your daily reality."

Discovering Your GoddessPleasure in the Divine Dimensions

As Esmerelda uses a drum to create a deep, steady beat every 4.5 seconds, Biss speaks in a soothing tone:

> My Goddesses, remember that the drum beat serves as a "sonic driver" to help you get into a trance-like state, and that it's been used by healers since ancient times. The beats "drive" your brainwaves into the Theta zone, which is just above a dream state and is the best way to connect with the infinite energy of the Universe. You can call this energy God, Goddess, Creator, Spirit, Source, your Higher Self or another term that resonates with your beliefs. I'm going to say Spirit during this meditation.
>
> Keep your eyes closed and your bodies still.
>
> First, let's set the intention to journey into the divine realms where we can connect with Spirit and learn what we need to know to get clarity on your

Tuesday, Day 3

GoddessPleasure Vision, along with the action steps that will open the gateway into your GoddessLife.

Let's begin by imagining a golden beam of light shooting down from the sky like a supernatural elevator shaft that will transport you into the spiritual dimensions.

You start this process with your imagination, but at some point, you'll transcend into a multi-sensory experience that doesn't feel like it's coming from your own mind. You may see, hear and encounter beings, ideas, spoken messages and visions that are unexpected or unfamiliar; this indicates that the information is coming from Spirit rather than your imagination. Listen, observe and allow the experience to unfold.

As the light beam surrounds you, call out to your spirit guide to escort you. This guide may show up as a powerful spiritual being such as the Egyptian Goddess Isis. An angel may wrap you in their wings. A unicorn may invite you to get on its back. An ancestor may take your hand. Your spirit animal may show up to guide you, symbolizing characteristics that you need to adopt, such as a lion teaching you courage, or an eagle showing you how to soar above the ordinary and look at the big picture.

In your mind, greet your spirit guide and thank them in advance for escorting you into the spiritual dimensions. Then state your intention: "Please show me the details of my GoddessPleasure Vision, what's blocking me from experiencing it, and the action steps I need to take to manifest it in my physical reality."

Next, allow your spirit-self to detach from your physical body and ascend up this beam with your guide. As you ascend, know that you are safe and surrounded by an army of angels. You may feel a floaty sensation. Keep going.

Just as an airplane passes through a layer of clouds as it ascends toward the infinity of sky and space, you also pass through a lavender veil that separates the divine dimensions and the physical world. So feel yourself gently floating upward, up, up—light as a feather—up this golden beam with your spirit guide, until you land in your "power spot," the unique space where you "land" upon arriving in the divine realms.

With your spirit guide at your side, know that this experience is different for everyone. There's no right or wrong. You may see, hear, feel or simply know new information that comes in the form of spoken words, images, feelings, symbols and scenes as if they're playing on a divine movie screen. Likewise, you may enter into a vivid world that looks like outer space, a garden, an enchanted forest or even a golden palace in the clouds. Be open to what you experience.

Next, ask Spirit: "Please show me my Goddess-Pleasure Vision, what's blocking me from experiencing it, and the action steps I need to take to manifest it in my physical reality."

You may see, feel, hear or sense a presence. The spiritual being or beings that show up to help you

Tuesday, Day 3

> may take you somewhere—to a throne, an altar, a forest, a floaty place in space, a house or anywhere. You may hear words, see symbols or be shown visions. Ask questions. Listen. When the interaction concludes, thank God and/or the angels and/or other beings who helped you.
>
> Now I'm going to give you some time to journey in the divine realm and learn what you need to know to bring your GoddessPleasure Vision to life.

Biss is silent while Esmerelda continues her drumming every 4.5 seconds. You and the women and silent and still as you journey in the spiritual dimensions. After 10 minutes, Biss resumes:

> It's time to thank the divine beings who showed up to help you. Make sure you imprint everything in your mind so you can remember it and write about it when you come out of meditation.
>
> With your spirit guide, make your way back to your power spot. From there, slide down the golden beam of light, ever so gently, floating like a feather in the breeze.
>
> Just as the airplane passes through the layer of clouds to return to earth, you pass through the lavender veil that separates the divine realms from the physical world. Then continue to float down like a leaf in the wind, down, down, back to yourself.
>
> Notice the stillness in your body and the slowness of your heartbeat and breathing. Slowly reacclimate to yourself by wiggling your fingers and toes. Take some deep breaths, and when you're ready, open your eyes.

What did Spirit tell you? Were your questions answered? Did you receive instructions? Notice how you feel now. Describe your experience in your *PowerJournal*. Make sure you record any action steps that Spirit provided to make your Goddess-Pleasure Vision real.

I'm going to give you 10 minutes to journal. You can also go back and fill in the Action Steps column of the GoddessPleasure Gateway Worksheet. Spirit will speak through this intuitive writing, so let it flow. Don't think about it or process it. Just keep writing until every detail is on the page.

After 10 minutes, Esmerelda makes a gong sound.

"Alright," Biss says, "who'd like to share what Spirit told you about activating your GoddessPleasure?"

Andi's hand shoots up. "Well, I take the cake for the most freaked out by this stuff, so please let me go first. Just like yesterday, Nell showed up. My spirit guide. My question was, *How the hell will know what to do with a woman in bed, if all I've done is fantasize about it, but I've never done it? What if I suck at it!?*"

"Then she'll like that," Jade says playfully as Andi and other women laugh. "Just like dudes do." Jade tells Biss, "Sorry for my crass humor."

"All good," Biss says as several women smile while others write in their journals, oblivious to the banter.

Andi anxiously runs her hand through her hair. "And I asked to see my vision for Pleasure, along with what's blocking me, and what I need to do to make it happen. And all of I sudden, I swear I felt dizzy and floaty, and I was in the beach house that I saw yesterday. It was like a continuation of that scene. My wife Billie and I finished the tacos that she made—they were so delicious!—and

Tuesday, Day 3

we got in the hot tub, laughing and kissing and wearing matching rings. And then—" Andi looks around, embarrassed "—I don't want to give the saucy details, but I had sex skills that my wife *loved!* I felt like a champ! And there was so much love, more love than I've ever felt in my life."

Biss smiles. "What did Nell say are your obstacles and what are your action steps?"

"Yeah," Andi says. "Nell said a couple things. First, I have to write out this scene, every detail, and read it out loud like you said. So it stays active in my mind. They said I also need to join this group that's for lesbians who come out late in life, for moral support and tips that will boost my confidence. And to find my wife, Nell said she's an artist and I'll meet her after I get my beach house-slash art studio in Provincetown. But I have to get myself situated first."

"That's what's up," Zeusse says.

"Provincetown is one of the most LGBTQ+ friendly places on the East Coast," Andi says, "and Nell told me I can easily find my tribe there and succeed as a queer-owned business." Andi's gray eyes grow wide. "Man, I am still freakin' out that this really works. Anybody else, I'd call bullshit and say you're talkin' a bunch of hocus pocus."

Several women laugh.

"Andi!" Biss smiles. "You're activating your GoddessPower and your GoddessPleasure. Thank you for sharing. I'm excited for you to experience all that Nell said and more."

"Me next!" Sammie says eagerly. "So the whole idea of activating *my* Pleasure is terrifying, because that's what's gotten me in trouble in the first place. And yesterday when the Egyptian queen showed up and told me don't date for a year so I can find my dream husband, I'm like, *Why am I even talking about Pleasure? That's gonna put me right back in ManLand!"*

"Uh, yeah!" Marla exclaims with a sarcastic tone.

"So in the meditation," Sammie continues, "I asked to see my GoddessPleasure Vision and what's blocking me and what I need to do. The queen showed up again, and she showed me my energy body, like you said Biss when we clear our chakras. But it was like this murky bubble around my body, and it was full of cloudy areas and splotches like dirt and stains, and she was like, these are the energy imprints from all your past lovers. Then there were these lines all through my energy body, scraggly lines like a kid had made them with a crayon, and they were giving off gray sparks."

All the women are looking at Sammie and listening intently. She flips her long straight yellow hair over a shoulder and says, "The queen told me, these crazy lines are neuron pathways or something like that, like ruts where my old thought patterns just keep getting stuck and repeating the same back-and-forth motion, like a car that's stuck in the mud." Her voice cracks. "She said my brain is literally programmed for this, because it's been my habit for years, and that my whole body craves the familiarity of this fucked-up thinking and behavior of chasing men who make me crazy! Even more twisted is that my entire being thinks this is Pleasure, but it's actually hurting me on every level."

"OhmyGod," Marla exclaims.

"Yeah, it's beyond fucked up." Sammie's eyes brim with tears.

"Did your spirit guide provide a solution?" Biss asks.

"Yeah, that's why I'm supposed to quit men cold turkey for a year," Sammie says. "To cleanse all those energy stains out of my system and erase those lines of thought patterns and behaviors, while I'm doing massive self-care and self-Pleasure, to purify myself."

"That's deep!" Zeusse says.

"I love that," Sunshine exclaims.

Sammie looks awed. "The Egyptian queen kept saying, 'Stay pure, dear one. Stay pure, dear one.'" She looks around at the women. "This shit is so real. I really think I can do this! And I can't wait to get all those toys in my tent tonight. I'm gonna need them!" She laughs and wipes her tears at the same time.

"Sammie," Biss says, "your spirit guide reminds us that when you're intimate with another person, their energy makes imprints on *your* energy body. And their soul carries the imprints of all their past partners. So if your lover is living a low-vibe lifestyle and having sex with other low-vibe people, then all that toxicity is brewing inside your lover like an energy storm that, during sex, thunders into your system, leaving you anxious and feeling bad."

Biss nods. "This also applies to same-sex partners, because it's about our energy bodies fusing during sex, regardless of what organs we're using."

The screen shows two people surrounded by energy bubbles—one pink, one purple—coming together. Their energy bubbles overlap, then the pink seeps into the purple and the purple seeps into the pink, creating one color that's a blend of both.

"This happens, even during the heat of attraction before you physically touch, and just gazing into the windows of each other's souls, your eyes," Biss says. "Then the energy fusion accelerates when you're touching and kissing; penetration with tongues, fingers and penises thrusts that energy inside the woman's body. So condoms can't protect you from STDs, Sexually Transmitted Demons."

"Gross!" Bianca scowls.

"And remember," Biss says, "if you don't use a condom, a man is literally injecting his DNA into your body. That's the goal if you want to have a baby. But if Pleasure is your singular goal, think about that. Aside from the health risks, do you want the DNA of a casual sex partner inside your body?"

"No!" Jade squirms on her sofa. "And didn't you say something yesterday about a 90-year-old woman who had sperm in her brain?"

Biss nods. "A study showed that male DNA was found in the brain of a 90-year-old woman. Which means the sperm had traveled through her body and lodged in her brain, probably decades ago."

Groans echo through the tent.

"My Goddesses," Biss says, "you have the freedom to have sex with whomever you want, and with as many people as you want. But when you learn about the energy exchange that happens during sex, and how it can drain and literally stain your energy with someone's toxicity—you can make informed decisions about whether it's worth it."

Jade raises her hand. "This makes me really glad I'm not hooking up with anyone right now. What we're learning is like the opposite of an aphrodisiac."

Biss smiles. "It's time to lavish yourself with love, and that, as Sammie just described, will prepare you on an energetic level to attract your sacred partner, if that's what you're seeking. Or, it will purify your energy to create the clearest connection to Spirit and put you in your optimum GoddessGenius Zone to build your empire."

"All that sounds heavenly to me," Sunshine says. "During my meditation, my grandmother came to me this time! She said she knows who my future husband is, and that he's looking for me, but he's doing the work on himself to heal just like I am. And that I need to work with the therapist to forgive my biological father for being a monster. I have to release my rage at him and my grief that his sexual violence killed my mother. Nani said those emotions are my blocks. She said I have to indulge myself with Pleasure in every

Tuesday, Day 3

way, every day, so that I can practice making myself believe that I'm worthy of receiving everything I desire in life."

"That's powerful," Biss says.

"Nani showed me my GoddessPleasure Vision," Sunshine says. "It was my wedding night, in an overwater bungalow in Fiji, in a big bed with white mosquito draping and tropical pink flowers everywhere. I was wearing the most beautiful lingerie and my husband was pleasuring me in a way that was better than anything I've experienced, because I felt so safe and free. I wasn't self-conscious about my body. I wasn't worried that he would ever cheat on me or hurt me. I knew in my core that he's mine and I'm his, forever—"

Sunshine buries her face in her hands and sobs. "I want this all like, yesterday."

Biss asks with a gentle tone, "Did your grandmother elaborate on your action steps to make your GoddessPleasure Vision your reality?"

"The same as yesterday," Sunshine says. "Therapy. Daily meditation, energy clearing and journaling. And a plant-based diet with no processed food or sugar. To cleanse my system."

"Beautiful," Biss says. "Sunshine and all of you, if you haven't already, please write down every detail from your meditations while it's fresh in your mind."

Zeusse raises her hand. "My grandmother came to me, too. It was the one in Alabama who shamed me. Mama G apologized to me! She said—" Zeusse pauses, then imitates her grandmother's Southern dialect "—'Baby, them was my human ways. Now up here in heaven, I see things different. It's all love. You go love who you wanna love. I was just scared for you, is all. Wanted to protect my precious lil' grandbaby girl. Not so lil' no more. Proud of you, girl. Your Mama G proud of you!'"

Zeusse wipes a tear with her fingertips. "Aw snap, I forgot. That angel from yesterday, Archangel Gabriel, escorted me to this pond in the woods by my grandparents's farm, where Mama G was sitting on a log, fishing and talking to me. She had on her favorite blue house dress, work boots, and a straw hat, and her skin was glowing like brown sunshine. And her eyes—they turned blue when she got old—they were beaming all this love toward me."

Everyone is quiet.

"Zeusse," Biss says, "did your grandmother show you a vision of your GoddessPleasure?"

Zeusse laughs and looks around. "Yawl, don't expect some Victoria's Secret-type answer from me. Mama G said go to my linen closet and pull out the old quilt she made me, you know the kind made outta patches from back in the day, all stitched together and heavy as hell?"

"Crazy quilts!" Celeste says. "I have three and wouldn't sell 'em for a million bucks. There's love and history in every stitch and patch of fabric from our people's clothes, curtains, you name it."

"Right," Zeusse says. "Mama G knew I *loved* sleeping under that quilt because at bedtime, I would run my fingers over all the satin and velvet and corduroy patches and she'd tell me a story about what she and Grandad did in the clothes that she'd cut up to make the quilts. They lived the glamorous life back during a time when that wasn't common for Black folks. But they had money to come to New York and go to formal events and what not, and I remember Mama G and Grandad looking so elegant and sharp when they stayed with me and Pops and went out on the town."

Zeusse looks up in happy reverie. "Anyway, Mama G said now I need to sleep under that quilt every night and touch the fabrics and feel the love she put into making it and remember the happy stories and the love she had with Grandad, and know I can find that someday, too. I never thought of a nostalgic quilt as Pleasure, but it makes sense."

Zeusse smiles, "Then, the icing on the cake, Mama G showed me and my boo under that blanket, all cuddled up and happy." She shakes her head. "I couldn't tell if she was my part-time boo that I want for now, or my forever girl. All I know is, this is some wild shit, for real."

Several women comment in agreement.

"Did she tell you any other action steps?" Biss asks.

"Yeah, she said I need to do more special things for myself every day. Like pick up a healthy meal instead of fast food. Buy some nicer dishes, silverware and towels. And make one of the bedrooms in my brownstone into a dope-ass office where I really dig working to make The Zeusse Girls Basketball Academy happen. Oh, and Mama G said think of Pleasure in every detail of my office. Get the bomb desk and CEO chair, make it smell like my favorite scent—sandalwood, display all my trophies and medals and favorite books in a lighted case, play my favorite beats by Janelle Monae and Frank Ocean, and get artwork and lighting that set the mood to stay in my power and work, not in a hype way, but in a zen flow state."

"Wow," Kiki says. "Sounds amazing."

Zeusse smiles.

"Thank you for sharing, Zeusse," Biss says.

"My turn!" Celeste exclaims. "My whole thing was about self-care. I'm already good with self-Pleasure and intimacy with my husband. Thank God for that! But self-care? Not so much. Hence, the oozing eczema that led me here. So, my Auntie Rose showed up again and said my GoddessPleasure goes hand in hand with my GoddessPower. Since baking brings me Pleasure, and sharing what I bake with people brings me Pleasure, my mission to open Celeste's Sweet Shop is all about Pleasure. But what I have to do, and what she showed me in my Vision, is that I have to incorporate Pleasure into my self-care, which has been a big fat zero for a long time."

"Same," Jade says.

"Auntie Rose showed me having a ball all by my damn self in my own private room in my house," Celeste says. "Right now, that room is a guest suite that we use for storage. It's a hot mess! But my action step is to change it into my own private sanctuary. It'll have plush furnishings like this—" she runs her fingers over the velvet sofa "—where I can sit and read. There's a massage table. And there's a desk where I can journal. There's a mini wine cooler and fridge for snacks. There's a little cove where I can sit and meditate. And the en suite bathroom is like a mini-spa just for me, for bubble baths and pampering."

"I want that, too!" several women exclaim.

"Do it!" Celeste says. "Auntie Rose said my blocks are that I put everyone's needs before mine. My kids, my husband, my parents who are in assisted living with dementia, my work. And there's nothing left for me by the time I collapse in bed at one in the morning. She said I have to use the GoddessPower Activation Tools to work on deserving. Feeling worthy of putting myself first. She said it's not selfish to put myself first. It's required. She told me to say, 'I deserve the best' to myself all day long, and to spend at least one hour every day, no matter how busy things get when I open the café, in Celeste's Sanctuary. She said the self-care and Pleasure will make my eczema a thing of the past, halleluiah."

Biss raises her arms in the air. "Everybody hear that? Self-care is GoddessPleasure!"

"Yes!" Bianca says.

Tuesday, Day 3

"I can't make this happen soon enough," Celeste says. "I'm submitting my resignation as CEO on Monday and I'll start looking for my commercial kitchen and creating my private room at home. Biss, I am so elated and grateful to be here. I haven't felt this excited in too damn long."

Biss beams a big smile at Celeste. "I'm honored to inspire that in you."

Marla raises her hand. "My GoddessPleasure Vision is giving me so much hope! I think I actually had an orgasm during the meditation. OhmyGod, I can't believe this. It was wild. Like this feeling that started between my legs and expanded out like little waves and my body twitched and my brain was like watching wild colors, like those little toys that kids look through and see moving shapes—"

"A kaleidoscope," Sammie says.

"Yeah!" Marla continues, "I was seeing a freaking kaleidoscope in my mind while my body had these rad sensations, and Lady Hope, the same spirit escort from yesterday, she like wrapped me in her arms and took me into three different rooms. In the first room, I was with myself, in my bedroom, making myself feel this way!"

Marla pauses to dab tissues to her eyes, slightly smudging her black eyeliner. "In the second room, I was with this beautiful man, I think he was my boyfriend and maybe fiancé, but it was a love scene that was better than anything I've seen in a movie, and the best thing was, I was having that rad feeling in my mind and body, with him! He was taking me there, and I had no blocks, no guilt, no shame!"

Sammie looks eager. "Third room? Tell us!"

"No sex in the third room," Marla says. "It was an all-white room and it was just me and my parents on two sofas, and like my extended family and our church community were all sitting in pews behind them, and I was on one sofa facing them all, and I literally think God was sitting beside me. It wasn't a person. It was like a gold cloud of electricity with—wow, this sounds so cray-cray—shooting stars and huge sparklers coming out of it and surrounding me, giving me a superpower to speak my mind to my parents and everybody, and I felt no fear as I said, 'I forgive you and I'm being true to me from now on,' and more of that gold energy came in me while these gray clouds sprayed out of me and my parents floated toward me in the best hug ever. Then they were flung back, and they and all the people became really small and I got bigger and bigger until I couldn't see them anymore and I was floating up—"

Marla stops herself and looks around. "I sound like I took ecstasy or something!"

"No, keep going!" Sammie orders. "This is better than watching Netflix."

"So when I floated up," Marla continues, "I was lighter and all those Pleasure feelings from the first two rooms were in me—she looks at Sammie—and it ended with *us!* Launching our skincare line with all new branding that Lady Hope says will come to us while we're here this week. Tomorrow, when we meditate on our GoddessProsperity."

"Yeah, bitch!" Sammie shrieks.

Sunshine gasps. "Oh, yes, yes, yes!"

Marla continues. "She said all the Ps here are connected, and you can't do one without the other."

"Beautiful," Biss says. "Marla, did Lady Hope give you action steps?"

"Yeah, it was the same as what she already said. I have to write in my journal that I forgive my parents and everybody else

Tuesday, Day 3

for every single thing that comes to mind, and I have to do this every day until I'm like, empty. And I have to write that I forgive myself for dwelling on all this and feeling so mad about it, so I can release it."

Marla pauses. "And Lady Hope said when I do this, it will open space inside me to let the Pleasure happen with myself and with the man or men I attract."

Biss smiles. "Yes! That has been my experience, and this echoes back on Sammie's vision and action steps to cleanse the toxic smudges from her energy field."

"I'm trippin' on all this," Zeusse tells Marla, "and I believe it."

Marla beams at Zeusse, then adds, "Oh, wait! Lady Hope told me I'll have three high value men who want me really bad, and that I'll get to choose which one I want."

"That's hot, girl!" Sammie says.

Bianca raises her hand. "My Vision was all about feeling safe around Pleasure. The giant dog, my spirit animal, took me into the coziest place, it wasn't really a room, it was a feeling, and there was this forcefield around me and I knew that nothing and no one could come through it to hurt me. I was alone, working on my girls center, and I was with the lover I have on call, and this angel was with us and said I'm safe with him and he's all I need for now."

She looks down and wipes tears from her eyes. "This lover is very gentle with me and very sensitive to my mobility. The angel told me to let him help me more, that I don't have to do everything alone. Like he's always offering to take me swimming in the ocean, but that terrifies me, even though before the accident, I used to feel total bliss in the ocean. I always tell him no, because I don't trust. The angel said I can trust him. My friend, Jonathan, said he would hold me and let me float and feel the warm salty water on my body and stare up at the blue sky and the hot sun on my skin—"

Bianca sobs. "I haven't done that since the accident. But I think about it every day when I stare out at the water from by balcony. I used to love to go over the bridge to Coronado Island and go to the beach there and just float for what felt like forever. The angel showed me doing that, with him—his name is Jonathan—holding me, and I'm trusting him to keep me safe."

She takes a deep breath. "He is also so loving with my body. How he kisses me and touches me and helps me orgasm. The angel told me to stop being self-conscious about my scars and limitations, and instead focus on the gratitude of being alive and able to enjoy Pleasure in so many ways. And that Jonathan is here for a season to prepare me for a forever partner who will be all that and more."

"Oh my God," Jade says softly. "That's like the best movie. I can see it so clearly."

"That's beautiful, Bianca." Biss smiles at her and looks at you and all the women. "My Goddesses, notice how Spirit is taking all of you out of your comfort zones, which were actually traps of discomfort where we stay because it's familiar."

"No more!" Andi says.

"Bianca, did the angel provide any specific action steps?" Biss asks.

"I have to practice Pleasure every day with myself," Bianca says. "Around food, drink, bathing, my bedtime routine, and what I see and hear every day. I have to make a list every morning of five things I'll do in each area to make sure I enjoy the sensual Pleasures of my life. And specifically for Jonathan, I have to invite him over for dinner and tell him that I'm open to receive his offers for things that I've declined in the past. Even a vacation in Cabo San Lucas in Mexico, where my grandparents still live. He offered to take me for a week, but I didn't want to go to a place where I'd

Tuesday, Day 3

see the beach and be too afraid to go in the water like I did as a kid every day when I visited my Grandma Carmen and Grandpa José. Now I'm ready."

Biss smiles at Bianca. "That is lovely, Bianca."

Kiki raises her hand. "So I don't want anything traditional. This was so rad, because I came here so lost and clueless about what to do with my life."

Kiki's dark eyes glow with awe. "The Hindu Goddess Lakshmi came and showed me my PleasureVision of opening a club that's kind of a sex club but super upscale, where people come to see erotic shows and meet people who don't want to live the vanilla life. Like people in open relationships or people who are ENM, Ethically Non Monogamous, or polyamorous or throuples—"

"What's that?" Andi asks.

"Three people in a committed relationship," Kiki says. "Like two men and a woman or two women and a man or three nonbinary people."

"I don't understand nonbinary," Sunshine says.

"It means people who don't identify as strictly male or strictly female, but somewhere in between," Kiki says. "The most important thing is that *they* get to define themselves. Got it?"

Sunshine nods. "Thank you."

Biss says, "Kiki, tell us more about your PleasureVision."

"The Goddess Lakshmi, she showed me in some kind of incubator for entrepreneurs, like a contest for start-ups, and I win the money to open the club. She told me a website where I can sign up when I get home. She said this will solve my fear and shame when I sneak around to hook up, because right now I'm financially dependent on my brother and his wife in Miami. When I have my own money, and success in business, I'll have the power to make my own decisions and do whatever the fuck I want, whenever, however, and with whoever I want."

"Hell yeah!" Sammie exclaims. "Bad ass bitches unite!"

Kiki smiles.

"So besides money," Biss says, "did Lakshmi identify any other blocks for you?"

"She said the forgiveness meditation with you will help me get rid of all my fucked up feelings toward my family," Kiki says, "because they're just trying to do what they think is best for me. I also have to forgive myself for so many years of hating myself for not figuring out what to do with my life. Lakshmi said I was *supposed* to wander through the fog, so when I find my way and open my club, I'll put everything in me into making it successful. And that doing it in Miami will be successful, because there's so many Pleasure-seeking people there who want to live the wilder life."

Biss smiles. "This is exciting for you, Kiki."

Kiki's eyes glaze with tears. "Biss, I've *never* had any kind of vision for my life. Or the confidence that I can actually do it."

"It's the magic of Infinity Mountain," Biss says, "and your Supernatural Self, revealing your truth. For all of you."

Kiki nods. "I have to write out every little detail about the club, inspired by my own fantasies. Like, the interior design. The shows. The wait staff. The signature drinks. The tables and stage and bar. The dress code and code of conduct. Security. Oh, and it's called Kinkee's. Like, my name plus kinky, with a fun spelling."

"We'll do a social media blow-up for you to promote it," Marla says. "With a VIP opening and we'll invite every influencer we know."

"Me and Marl!" Sammie says. "And models. You need sexy food like we have here in the Pleasure Tent. A menu of aphrodisiacs!"

"You're all ahead of the game," Biss says. "You just described tonight's GoddessFeast. Kiki, anything else to share?"

"Yeah. In my personal life, I'll be as wild and freaky and kinky as I want. Kiki can finally fly her freak flag, loud and proud. Nothing

Tuesday, Day 3

traditional for me. Like, *ever*. I want to date couples and make a sex room in my own house when I can buy one, and go to swingers parties and nudist resorts and sex cruises, and just explore everything."

Several women express surprise and say, "I've never heard of any of that!"

Biss tells Kiki: "I applaud your courage to live and love as you truly desire. Just always put safety first."

"I do now," Kiki says. "And I'll keep doing that. I have a guy friend who goes to parties with me. I hate that I like, need a bodyguard, but I know that's smart. I never set down my drink or let anybody hand a drink to me, so they can't spike it. I also don't drink or get high when I'm out."

"Smart," Biss says. "Anything else, Kiki?"

"Biss, I can't remember feeling this clear on things, or excited about my future. Usually, I wake up in the morning feeling like such a fucking loser. Thank you." She starts crying, and Sammie hops onto her sofa and hugs her.

Jade raises her hand. "I'm more like Kiki and Bianca. I don't want a real relationship. I like having a few lovers to call on when I'm in the mood. Plus, when my band starts traveling a lot, I don't want to be tied down to a relationship. Me and a girl in my band, sometimes we hook up or pick up a dude together. So I'm good on that."

Biss nods. "Tell us about your PleasureVision."

"Well like yesterday," Jade says, "it started off fuzzy. Like I couldn't get on the beam, and nobody showed up as my spirit guide. But then all of a sudden, I heard a motorcycle and Ellie roared in! It was so freaking cool. She said 'Let's go!' and I was on her motorcycle going straight up. It was scary, but more fun than any rollercoaster. And then we were like whizzing around the whole world, over and over, with cities lighting up like stars, and she was talking too fast for words; I just knew what she was telling me, and she named every major city in Europe and Asia, Africa, Australia, South America and North America."

Jade looks ecstatic. "Then Ellie took me to one of our concerts. The Star Chix were playing in Tokyo. And I was on stage playing my guitar for a packed arena. All these guys and girls were going crazy when I was playing my new songs and I could see myself on stage. Orange and red light was glowing around me, like see-through flames, and Ellie said that was the creative energy of my sacral chakra and the money power of my root chakra, because I'm making a shit-ton of money from my music and tours, and that the orange-red light was also showing that I was in my ultimate Pleasure zone—on stage, performing."

"Did Ellie tell you what's blocking you and what action steps you need to take?" Biss asks.

"She said be patient," Jade says. "I'm supposed to go home and write my new songs and save as much money as possible and work with our promoter to set up local shows and get my new song played on the radio. And that will make everything explode. So the blocks are my impatience and procrastination and negative thinking and the stuff with my parents. And the action steps are to write songs and practice six days a week, and like immerse in the Pleasure of my creativity. And I have to make peace with my parents, not talking about the tough stuff yet, just like going to dinner and warming up to them."

"How are you feeling about that?" Biss asks.

"I'm okay with it," Jade says, "because if that's what it takes to get me into my GoddessLife, then I'm game for anything."

"You can do it," Biss says.

Delaney raises her hand. "My spirit guide, the lady on the white horse, showed me my PleasureVision. It was very similar to yesterday, so at first, I thought I was making my mind replay my meditation in the Pyramid. I was feeling immense peace and again floating in a warm, watery cocoon, but this time, the lady on the white horse was saying, 'Delaney, you are enough,' and her words flowed into my body with waves of orgasm. She said, 'Your GoddessPleasure is in cultivating self-love so deeply that it brings you to orgasm.'"

Delaney looks around nervously. "I feel quite embarrassed sharing something so personal."

"You're safe here," Biss says.

"And I feel guilty, because I don't want to sound like this is against my husband," Delaney says. "My spirit guide said it's all about me. And the blocks are guilt over the idea of separating my needs from my husband's needs, along with the grip that my mother still has on my perception of myself. So the action steps are to work the GoddessPleasure Activation Tools every day to find myself, while knowing that loving and caring for myself doesn't mean loving my husband any less."

Delaney pauses, pushing her silver curls behind one ear. "And that I'm free to replace the negative aspects of my mother's influence with gratitude that she raised me and everything formed me into who I am today."

"Beautifully said," Biss says.

Delaney nods. "Thank you."

Biss looks at you and says, "Would you like to share next?"

Welcome to The Biss Tribe

Dear Goddess Reader:

Please describe your meditation experience, including: your encounter with your Spirit Guide; what happened in the divine realm; what you learned about your GoddessPleasure Vision; what's blocking you; and what specific action steps you need to take to bring it into reality.

_____

_____

_____

_____

_____

_____

A Healing Meditation to Release Shame, Guilt, Fear and Trauma Around Your Sexuality

The Concierges serve you and each woman smoothies of your choice: peanut butter and green apple, coconut-pineapple-macadamia, banana-strawberry-walnut, and a three-berry Greek yogurt blend. You sip your smoothie from a beautiful crystal goblet, enjoying the cold flavors and thick, creamy texture.

"This is the bomb," Zeusse says. "I need to get back into my smoothie groove every day."

"Yeah," Jade says, "I should have this instead of ice cream every night. Ellie told me that numbing out on sugar shuts down my creativity."

Tuesday, Day 3

Andi nods. "I used to think that M&Ms helped me paint, but I get a sugar high and crash into massive brain fog."

"My café at The Turquoise Experience," Sunshine says, sipping her green apple and peanut butter smoothie, "will have meals that are specifically crafted to give you sustained energy. You have to combine protein, healthy fats, and slow-burn carbs like brown rice and quinoa every time you eat. So the energy is released slowly. Cheers." She holds up her glass toward Andi, who does the same back.

"My Goddesses," Biss says, "these smoothies will keep you hydrated and energized as we embark on this next and very important meditation. We're going to call on the healing angel, Archangel Raphael, to do a healing around any shame, guilt, fear and trauma you may have around your sexuality. This metaphysical healing can change you on the cellular level, as well as remove emotional and psychological wounds that are blocking you from enjoying your GoddessPleasure."

The word "forgiveness" appears on the screen above Biss. "Let's talk about forgiveness. It's actually the act of healing *yourself* by releasing painful feelings, emotional wounds and oppressive programming that someone else inflicted on you. In fact, the Merriam-Webster dictionary defines 'to forgive' as: 'to cease to feel resentment against' an offender. Forgiveness is an inside job! It's a shift in feelings."

"This is hard," Sunshine says. "I've tried to forgive my biological father. The 48-year-old married man who raped my mother when she was 13 then died in childbirth with me. The whole forgiveness thing just never worked for me. I just feel rage toward him and the world about it. He threatened to kill my family if they went to the police, so he was never prosecuted and got to keep living his life. I resent him beyond words."

Biss casts a sympathetic look at Sunshine and says, "That's understandable. Consider this. Nelson Mandela once said: 'Resentment is like drinking poison and then hoping it will kill your enemies.'"

"That's exactly it," Sunshine says, "because I feel sick to my stomach when I think about him."

Biss continues: "If you don't forgive someone, it only hurts you more, long after the offense was committed. Forgiveness is a major tenet of spirituality. But how do you do it? When it comes to our sexuality, and if it involves emotional or physical trauma, it can be extremely difficult."

Bianca raises her hand. "Biss, can I share something?"

"Of course."

Tears glisten in Bianca's eyes. "When I was in college, I was raped in my dorm room by my boyfriend, who was an honors student. I was a virgin and I had told him no so many times." She wipes her eyes with tissues. "After that happened, it made me so terrified that every guy would assault me. And now that I'm in my chair, I'm even more vulnerable. I felt safe with my husband, but when he left me after the accident because I can't have babies, that made me feel unsafe to love again. I don't know if I can forgive either one of them—"

"Miraculous healings and forgiveness are possible," Biss says. "This meditation will begin the process."

"But I've carried the rape anger for almost 30 years," Bianca says. "Even worse was that the campus police and the city police told me it wasn't rape because he was my boyfriend and I let him into my room at night. And I was wearing a mini skirt and we were drinking. Classic victim-blaming."

"Horrible," Sunshine says as several women groan.

"They added insult to injury," Andi says. "That's so unfair, man."

Tuesday, Day 3

Biss casts a loving gaze at Bianca. "I know you can forgive, because I forgave a man who terrified me when I was five years old. Do you want to hear the story?"

The women say yes. Biss looks somber as she tells the story and Esmerelda continues her music:

> I was five years old, and all I wanted to do was play outside until my family was ready to leave for the funeral. It was a warm summer evening. I walked around our front yard, past the sandbox and blue plastic swimming pool. I didn't dare get wet or dirty—not in my new dress, black patent leather shoes, and white lace anklet socks. And I didn't want to mess up my hair; my mother had just styled my ringlets into two ponytails. Now she was doing my sister's hair while our father got dressed.
>
> As I stood on our corner lot, the teenaged brother of one of our playmates showed up, and lured me into their run-down house nearby. Suddenly I found myself in their bathroom, where he laid me on my back on the wet, dirty floor.
>
> My heart hammered with terror. I thought, *I have to get out of here!*
>
> I looked around. There was a bathtub, and—
>
> A giant knife glimmering on the sink! Panic shot through me.
>
> "My mommy's calling me!" I cried. She was not calling me; she didn't even know I was there.
>
> *Joey's brother is gonna chop me up and kill me!*
>
> "My mommy's calling me!" I cried.
>
> He lifted my legs up in the air.
>
> *God please don't let him kill me!*

My dress fell, exposing my panties and thighs. With eyes wide with fear, I looked up at my black patent leather shoes and white lace anklet socks. How could I escape?

"My mommy's calling me!"

I don't know if I knew what rape was, but I knew about intercourse. It was for grown-ups who were in love. This was not how it was supposed to happen. Nor was it something for kids. So whatever this guy was thinking was really bad.

"My mommy's calling me! Please let me go home! My mommy's calling me!"

I imagined my parents coming outside to get me, so we could go to the funeral. But they would not find me. And they might never know where I was. I had seen news reports about people killing kids and throwing the bodies in the river or in the woods. No! I had to escape!

Time seemed to drag on forever.

"Please let me go! My mommy's calling me!"

What was he going to do? He did not remove his clothes, nor did he touch me.

Finally, he let me leave.

I ran home. Terrified, horrified, relieved.

But silent. I didn't tell anyone what happened. I was sure that my father would storm over there and kill the guy. Then he would go to prison, and I wouldn't have a father.

So I said nothing. I just went home, thanking God for saving my life, while simultaneously replaying those terrifying moments when that guy could've done terrible things to me, snuffed out

Tuesday, Day 3

my young life, hidden my body, and left my parents with an unsolved mystery for life.

After the funeral, we visited my aunt and uncle's house. I went in the bathroom. From my vagina I pulled something with a sort of peanut skin consistency, only crispier; it was clear and amber brown. Maybe it was cockroach wings. Maybe on that nasty floor, a roach crawled into my panties, and its wings were my disgusting souvenir.

I left the bathroom and joined my family in the living room. And I said nothing about what the neighbor had done. But the heart-pounding terror replayed in my mind over and over and over that night when I went to bed—and *every* night for the rest of my childhood.

The tent is silent.

"Years later," Biss says, "during meditation, the guy came to me in spirit form and apologized. He had died long ago, a victim of street life. He said he was now working to protect other children. I said, 'I forgive you.' It wasn't about him. It was about me releasing the anger and fear that he had caused."

Bianca asks, "Did that make you afraid to date men?"

"Yeah," Andi asks, "did it interfere with you being able to enjoy sex?"

"Not directly," Biss says. "It just made me extra cautious about my safety. Years later, my therapist helped me see that as a little five-year-old girl, I was flexing GoddessPower, because my pleas convinced the guy to let me go without physically hurting me. So now when I think of that experience, I stay in gratitude that I survived, and see it from the perspective that I'm a strong bad ass survivor, even as a little girl."

The screen above Biss says, "Forgiving = Releasing."

She says, "So during my year-long retreat, where I did a lot of healing meditations and journaled about it, I learned how to heal and release hurtful experiences from this life and past lifetimes."

A few women groan.

"I don't know if I believe in reincarnation," Delaney says.

"That's okay," Biss continues. "Just know that forgiveness is a gift that we give ourselves. It has nothing to do with the other person. They don't even know that we may have spent years seething or hurting or ruminating about what they said or did, even if they had committed a terrible act. And even if it has blocked our Pleasure for a lifetime. Until now."

The women are silent as Esmerelda hits a woeful note in her wordless song and strokes a bowl to make a deep sound that reverberates through the tent.

"Oftentimes," Biss says, "people such as narcissists are so self-consumed with greed and oblivion to their hurtful, selfish ways, they're unaware and unconcerned about how they traumatize people. Even if it's criminal. So dwelling on them and wishing they would apologize or change or repent is pointless. It's better to go no contact and pour love into yourself."

Biss points up at the screen, which glows purple around the word "forgiveness" as she says, "Healing is all about **you.** Period. It's our responsibility to forgive. I'm not saying *excuse.* I'm saying release the emotional burden of dwelling on the hurts that someone caused. Forgiveness can also be applied to yourself."

Marla shakes her head. "No! I don't think I need to forgive myself. I'm the victim of all these people's brainwashing."

Biss nods. "Consider this. In the past, I've forgiven myself for wasting precious time and energy ruminating over someone else's hurtful words or actions. *They* did the damage, but *I* wasted time

Tuesday, Day 3

brooding about it, letting it distract me from being happy. Marla, do you see the point?"

"Yeah," she says. "I don't like it, but it's true. But how did you stop?"

"Journaling, meditation and therapy helped me process and expel this baggage from my mind," Biss says. "There is no shame in speaking with a therapist or trusted counselor, to help you unravel the thoughts and emotions so that you can release them and free your mind, body and spirit of the blocks. It's *not* easy. But it *is* possible."

Marla raises her hand. "Biss, I kind of think there might be something even deeper about my blockages around sex. Like, something I don't even know."

"That's the perfect segue into my next point."

The screen shows the image of a sad woman with cloudy shadows around her. Biss looks at you and all the women. "You may have blocks to your Pleasure that are caused by agreements or traumas in past lives. Remember yesterday—" she gazes at Marla "—after meditation when Marla, you said that Lady Hope told you that you had been a cloistered nun in a past life and that the vow of chastity that you had taken was still imprinted on your soul and affecting you in this life."

Marla nods and says, "Right. And to break free, I have to forgive my parents, which I still don't understand how to do."

"I'll show you," Biss says.

Andi sounds amazed: "This is also like yesterday in the Meditarium when Nell told me that dying in prison because I was gay in a past life, put a blueprint on my soul that made things play out in this lifetime until I find the courage to escape the blueprint." She laughs. "Man, if I had heard somebody say that just last week before I came here, I woulda said, 'Lady, you are *nuts!*'"

Welcome to The Biss Tribe

Andi's face glows with revelation. "Talk about a lightbulb moment. Man!"

Biss smiles. "I had a similar experience where a promise in a past life was blocking my Pleasure in this lifetime. Years ago, when I desperately wanted a lover, but felt very alone and self-isolating, Spirit revealed to me in meditation that in a past life, I had been a Catholic nun and had taken a vow of chastity. Just like Marla, that vow was still imprinted on my soul, and carried into this life, blocking me from finding a lover and having sex."

"So this is a common thing?" Marla asks.

Biss nods. "Yes, with any spiritual commitment you make in a past life. Tomorrow at the GoddessTreasure Cave, we'll talk about how vows of poverty taken in past lives by nuns or monks or others, can cause lack and financial struggles in this lifetime."

Many women groan as Zeusse asks, "How do you escape that?"

"Through healing meditations," Biss says. "For example, I asked Archangel Raphael to remove the vow of chastity that was still imprinted on my soul. The healing meditation allowed me to nullify the spiritual commitment and remove the block for me to attract a lover. It worked, because after the healing meditation, I stepped through GoddessPleasure Gateway into a whole new level. The most important take-away from that, my Goddesses, is that I had no idea that a vow made hundreds of years ago was robbing me of Pleasure in this life. And I only learned about it because I asked Spirit in meditation."

The screen shows two words:

*Medi-**c**-ation.*
*Medi-**t**-ation.*

"Let's talk about the healing power of meditation," Biss says. "Look at the words 'meditation' and 'medication.' Notice how only one letter is different: medi-c-ation and medi-t-ation. I believe these words are one and the same, because meditation can heal you emotionally, physically and spiritually."

The screen says: *"Disclaimer: I am not a physician. If you have a serious mental health condition or medical condition, please continue with your doctor's prescribed medical regimen."*

Biss glances up. "I'm about to guide you through a meditation that has healed debilitating physical pain—including migraine headaches and back pain—with no medication. It really works."

She looks at you and all the women. "And this healing experience can help remove anything that's obstructing, delaying or derailing your Pleasure. Plus, meditation can help you find inner peace, elevate into your creative GoddessGenius Zone, sleep better, lower your blood pressure, boost your mood, amplify your intuition, heighten your five physical senses, and make you have bigger, better, longer orgasms."

"Then let's get to it!" Kiki says playfully as several women cheer.

"So are you ready to experience the *PowerJournal for Forgiving and Healing with Archangel Raphael* technique to remove your blocks around Pleasure?"

"Yes!" Bianca exclaims as women cheer.

"We're going to call upon Archangel Raphael, who is non-denominational and all-loving," Biss says as the image of a giant angel aglow in emerald-green light appears on the screen.

"Angels are not human and do not have genders," she says. "The most powerful angels—known as archangels—include Archangel Raphael and are all about spiritual power that is bigger than the doctrine of a single religion. They are always available for you to call on their power to protect, heal and manifest."

On the screen, video shows beautiful angels whose enormous wings flutter and sparkle.

"You also have at least one guardian angel who has been with you since birth," Biss says. "You can get silent and still and ask them in your mind to reveal their name and signs of their presence in your life."

Biss smiles as "GoddessPower" appears on the screen.

"As I've said, the 'powers that be' haven't wanted the masses of humanity or women especially to know that we have access to the supernatural power of the Universe—to heal, receive psychic guidance and conceive innovative ways to do bold, brave things in the world. This is our GoddessPower! And part of that is our GoddessPleasure!"

An image of Archangel Raphael reappears on the screen.

"So," Biss continues, "back to our healing with Archangel Raphael, who will perform alchemy to transform negative emotions into Peace and Power. Let's get started. In your *PowerJournal*, find the page that says, 'Forgiving and Healing with Archangel Raphael.'"

As the sounds of turning pages fill the tent, Biss says, "Every person's healing meditation is different. There is no right or wrong way. Mine, for example, sometimes include Indigenous medicine men, as well as wolves and bears, which have medicinal powers. And I find myself suspended in the air as Archangel Raphael performs the healing. Just be open to what you experience."

Esmerelda's soothing music takes a more uplifting tone while Biss gives instructions for you to follow in your *PowerJournal*. She says:

> For the heading, write on the blank lines the name of the person or people who have blocked your GoddessPleasure, then write what you need to forgive them for, and what exactly you need to

Tuesday, Day 3

heal within yourself. Write today's date and location, which is The GoddessPleasure Tent.

PowerJournal to Forgive _____

and Heal _____

Date _____

Location _____

Then set your intention for this meditation.

My intention is to ask Archangel Raphael for a healing to forgive _____ *for* _____ *so that I can heal and release shame, guilt and fear, and replace those feelings with Peace and Power to experience my ultimate GoddessPleasure.*

My intention is also for Archangel Raphael to identify and remove any hidden blocks to my GoddessPleasure, and to help me forgive myself for allowing any thoughts, feelings or behaviors to sabotage my GoddessPleasure.

Describe how you'll feel after you've healed and released any blocks to your GoddessPleasure.

_____

_____

_____

_____

"After the meditation," Biss says, "you'll write about what happened with Archangel Raphael and what action steps you need to take to make GoddessPleasure one of the five foundations of your daily GoddessLife."

Biss points up at the screen, which says, "Gratitude helps you manifest."

"Now before we do this," she says, "know that it's extremely powerful to give thanks for something before it has happened. This demonstrates your faith that God/Spirit/Higher Self will divinely orchestrate circumstances to answer your prayer, according to your request or with something even better."

Dear Goddess Reader:

If you'd rather listen to Biss guiding you through this healing meditation, please use this QR code:

Tuesday, Day 3

Biss sits on her purple cushion and speaks in a soothing tone:

> Let's start by taking several deep breaths. Sit with your spine straight. You can also lie down, but not if you think you might fall asleep.
>
> Close your eyes. Become aware of any tension in your body and imagine your muscles softening like warm butter.
>
> Then envision a huge sunbeam, the kind you see shooting down from the sky through the clouds that look so majestic, especially around sunset when they glow with golden light. In your mind, call out to your spirit guide, who will escort you into the spiritual dimensions for this healing.
>
> Imagine that you, with your spirit guide at your side, are ascending this golden beam like a helium balloon in the breeze. See and feel yourself gently rising, ever so lightly, going up, up, up. You may feel a flutter in your stomach and a lightness of being. Just keep floating upward, knowing you are safe and surrounded by angels for as far as you can see.
>
> Ponder your intention to forgive a specific person as you ascend into a higher dimension where you're free to receive a healing with Archangel Raphael. Imagine yourself floating up this beam as if it's an elevator powered by pure love and Peace.
>
> As you ascend, you'll reach the lavender veil that separates the physical dimensions from the spiritual realms. This veil is similar to the layer of clouds that an airplane passes through as it ascends toward the infinity of sky and space. Above the veil, continue to float up. Soon you'll reach your "pow-

er spot" in the spiritual realm. This is your unique space where you're free to acclimate to this experience, then journey through divine dimensions to connect with Archangel Raphael.

You may experience this spiritual dimension as an enchanted forest, a mountainside, an Atlantis-type underwater wonderland, a rocky terrain, a golden palace, or something else. Simply observe what you hear, see and feel. Your spirit guide will remain with you. You are safe, surrounded by flocks of angels.

Next, allow your Supernatural Self to call out to Archangel Raphael, whom you may see, feel or simply know that they are present. God's healing angel performs healings amidst the emerald-green light of the heart chakra, which symbolizes pure love. So you may notice flashes of emerald green, or you may see a giant angel or the outline of wings. You may also simply feel the presence of a loving being.

Express your intention to forgive a specific person and/or yourself. And ask Archangel Raphael to reveal your blocks and remedies for removing them.

Archangel Raphael may take you to a particular place or lay you on a bed as if a medical procedure will be performed. Other beings may appear.

Since the Divine communicates through metaphors, you may see that Archangel Raphael is removing an object that represents the offense for which you're seeking forgiveness. For example, if you want to forgive someone for words and actions that instilled a lifetime of shame around your sexuality, Archangel Raphael may pull a slimy net from your body, symbolizing how that negative emotion had permeated your entire being.

This energetic "surgery" may also result in Archangel Raphael pulling cloudy globs of energy from you. Every healing meditation with Archangel Raphael is different, depending on the nature of the ailment. Sometimes, no physical object is removed.

Archangel Raphael's healing power is all about transmutation. In physics class, we learned the Law of Conservation of Energy: Energy can be neither created nor destroyed. It simply changes form. So Archangel Raphael takes the energy that's hurting you and transmutes or transforms it into healing energy. This happens as the angel removes your affliction and puts it in the lavender flame of St. Germaine that activates metaphysical alchemy. The lavender flame may appear as a shallow gold cauldron of vibrant purple fire.

When Archangel Raphael removes the symbol of toxic energy from your body—such as a slimy net, for example—and drops it into the lavender flames, the ailment/net crackles as the fire transforms it into healing energy. The slimy net burns away and takes the form of golden sparkles and emerald-green mist, which shoot up from the lavender flames in a great surge of golden sparks. Archangel Raphael then guides that golden healing energy to arc all around you and through you, filling your energy body with this powerful healing light.

You may feel a tingly sensation as this sparkling gold light permeates your entire being, entering your cells and infusing your psyche with love and peace where fear, guilt and shame once festered.

"It is done," Archangel Raphael declares, indicating that your healing is complete.

Thank the angel and listen for instructions, which could include praying, journaling, having direct communication with someone in the physical world, engaging in acts of gentle self-care, and taking action steps to continue your acts of forgiveness and healing to manifest your GoddessPleasure.

Make a point to remember everything that Archangel Raphael tells you, so that you can write it in your *PowerJournal* after the meditation. These will be your instructions to continue your passage through your GoddessPleasure Gateway.

Next, your spirit guide will return you to your power spot and escort you down the golden beam, ever so gently, like a feather in the breeze. And just like the airplane passes through the layer of clouds to return to earth, you pass through the lavender veil that separates the divine dimensions and the physical world. Float gently down, down, back to your body. Savor this deeply relaxed, peaceful state of being, and know that you can call upon the healing powers of Archangel Raphael anytime.

Now, wiggle your fingers and toes to re-acclimate to your body. I'll give you 10 minutes to write as many details as you remember. As you journal in this meditative state, you have a clear connection to Spirit. So ask questions in your mind and write the answers that Spirit provides, even if they seem fantastical. This Intuitive Writing should feel effort-

Tuesday, Day 3

less as Spirit speaks through your pen. Do not stop to analyze, just let the ideas flow freely.

Dear Goddess Reader:

Write about your healing meditation with Archangel Raphael. Describe what happened, what blocks were revealed, and what action steps you need to take to manifest your GoddessPleasure Life.

_____

_____

_____

_____

If you received any new action steps to manifest your GoddessPleasure, please write them in the third column of your GoddessPleasure Gateway worksheet.

After 10 minutes, Esmerelda sounds her gong.

"If you need to keep writing," Biss says, "please do. Would anyone like to share your experience with Archangel Raphael?"

Sammie, who's still sitting beside Marla, timidly raises her hand, looking around nervously. "This is super embarrassing. But my spirit guide said I have to share it to give all of you courage."

Biss nods with an encouraging expression. "We're here for you."

"Since my problem has been my man addiction," Sammie says, "and the solution is being celibate for a year," she pauses with reddening cheeks, "I'm supposed to make myself cum at least four times a week. Archangel Raphael showed me those same fucked up stains and lines in my energy, like the earlier meditation, but it was worse! They were like zigzags glowing crazy colors and short-circuiting all through me!"

Marla puts her arm around Sammie.

"I have to install new circuits," Sammie says. "That's what Archangel Raphael said. That pleasuring myself will rewire me energetically, so I'm not relying on guys for orgasms. When the angel put all the lines and stains in the fire, my whole system was clean. Then this big sparkly gold line formed from the top of my head down to my orange and red chakras—"

Sammie shoots a hard look at the women around her. "This is so hard. I'm trusting all of you to never tell a soul. My chakras all lit up really bright and the colors like exploded all through me. But Archangel Raphael said I won't stay that way unless I literally rewire myself through self-Pleasure and no men."

"That's the shit!" Marla exclaims. "Mine wasn't that clear. But it was similar."

"Sammie," Biss says, "thank you for sharing and I assure you, you have our strictest confidence."

Sammie looks down and starts writing.

"Marla, do you want to share?" Biss asks.

"Not really," Marla says. "It's too embarrassing."

"I'll go," Sunshine says. "Archangel Raphael pulled bloody barbed wire out of my entire body. It was so disgusting. My grandmother, who was a healer in the Navajo Nation, she was with him, and the energy around her was so bright, it was like the sun was behind her, shooting beams in every direction that felt hot while Archangel Raphael was surrounded by Indigenous healers. They were chanting and making all colors of light swirl around me to

Tuesday, Day 3

help Archangel Raphael pull the pain out of my body, which took a while, because it was so intertwined with every fiber of my being."

Sunshine wipes her eyes with tissues as her voice trembles: "The angel told me, 'You have to pray on forgiveness and healing every day.' After the bloody barbed wire burned up in the purple fire, and came back into my body as gold sparkles, my whole body twitched in the meditation and right here on this sofa. I could feel the change. I felt really hot sitting here, and I was shaking, and I heard the angel say, 'It is done.' And my grandmother raised her arms and my mother appeared and she was so beautiful and glowing with love and she said, 'My baby girl child, you are safe and so powerful. My death created the life of you. Give only love toward the seed of your father who created you in me.'"

Sunshine sobs so hard, her whole body moves up and down. Zeusse gracefully slides onto her sofa and says, "May I?"

Sunshine sobs into Zeusse's shoulder as Zeusse gently embraces her. The tent is silent except for women sniffling as Esmerelda plays her soothing song.

After a few minutes, Sunshine sits up and nestles under Zeusse's long arm. "My mother told me that this healing will free me to finally find my self-worth and build my business and be very successful at helping people find their purpose. Money will come. And my healing will raise me to a higher frequency where I can attract my husband."

"Beautiful," Biss says with a gentle tone.

"You good?" Zeusse says, casting a caring look down at Sunshine, who nods and says, "Yes, thank you so much."

"I got you," Zeusse says, then returns to her sofa.

"Thank you, Sunshine," Biss says, "and Zeusse. Would anyone else like to share?"

"That's a tough act to follow," Andi says. "Suffice to say for me that it worked and I know what I have to do."

"Same," Marla says.

Jade raises her hand. "Archangel Raphael told me exactly what to say to my parents, how to say it, and where. I wrote it all down. I can do this!"

Biss smiles. "Excellent."

"I had trouble at first," Bianca says. "When I hear healing, my question is, 'Can it make me walk again?' I've read books about how people have used spiritual healing and the power of the mind to reverse paralysis. But it's never worked for me. So I asked Archangel Raphael about it, and they said technology is being developed that can help me. But for now, the healing was all about forgiving the rapist, the drunk driver, and my ex-husband."

Bianca glances up with tears glistening in her eyes. "It's so hard. But in the meditation, I saw it. Those three men were like horror show bobble heads stuck in my body like mummified faces covered in bubbling slime. They were floating inside me, bumping around, taking up space, weighing me down. And laughing in a wicked way."

Delaney wipes her eyes as she watches Bianca speak.

"Archangel Raphael pulled them out," Bianca says. "And dropped them in the fire, and they were like gasoline on the flames, which got really big and hot, then turned into a gold plume, which the angel pushed back into me and said I have to journal every day for a week about forgiving those three men for every offense, and I have to write in my journal that I forgive myself for any negative self-talk I've had as a result."

"Powerful," Biss says. "Remember that forgiveness doesn't mean forgetting. It's important to remember what caused the need for forgiveness; those incidents helped form who we are.

We survived them. They made us stronger. And we have the divine right to thrive!"

Bianca wipes her eyes and nods.

Biss says, "You can all do this, Goddesses, because *you* have the Power!"

The Power of Pleasure: The Fifth GoddessPleasure Activation Tool

After a break for stretching and going to the restroom, you and the women return to your sofas, where the Concierges serve snacks on gold trays. Each offers an assortment of bite-sized wraps inspired by cuisines around the world: shawarma, pot stickers, dumplings, lettuce wraps, burritos, egg rolls, spring rolls, crepes, and naan with chutney.

"Ladies," Esmerelda says, "enjoy these samplings that are a global fusion of flavors. You can cleanse your palate between each bold flavor by dipping the tiny gold spoon into the little cup of sherbet."

"I love this," Sunshine says, gazing at the tray that also holds a plate of chocolates, nuts and colorful fruit arranged like flowers.

Sexy music plays and the dancers return to the stage around Biss as she says, "My Goddesses! Now that we've done the heavy lifting, it's time for the juicy stuff. Who's ready for that?"

"Yes!" Jade and Kiki exclaim as the women cheer.

"There's a fifth GoddessPleasure Activation Tool," Biss says. "Can anyone guess what it is?"

Kiki raises her hand. "I hope it's lots of sex."

"Close," Biss says. "It's self-Pleasure and the sensual indulgences that you can enjoy every day."

"So it's not just sex," Kiki says.

Welcome to The Biss Tribe

"It's much more," Biss says. "It starts with sensual Pleasure. This is anything that delights your senses, and what you see, hear, feel, taste, smell and sense through your intuition. Many of these things are already part of your everyday life, but prior to now, you may have overlooked them because you were too busy whizzing through the day, multitasking and letting worries to consume your thoughts. No more!"

The screen says: "Micro-Moments of Sensual Pleasure."

Biss continues: "I want you to enjoy micro-moments of sensual Pleasure every day. This will raise your vibration into the high-frequency emotions that help your Supernatural Self work her magic as you build your empire."

A woman on the far right asks, "What if you're asexual?"

Biss nods. "Great question. If you're asexual, which means you have no interest or desire for sex, you can still enjoy Pleasure in nonsexual ways, through the other senses. The beauty of GoddessPleasure is that *you* decide what you want and how you want it. So here are examples of nonsexual Pleasure that create micro-moments of happiness for me every day." Biss looks up at the screen and reads:

- Blissing out sunbathing in a thong bikini.
- Enjoying my morning coffee ritual.
- Snuggling into my sleep experience amidst the soft textures of flannel sheets, blankets and pillows.
- Massaging my feet with lavender oil before bed.
- Smelling essential oils while I'm working at my desk.
- Looking at and touching my colorful crystal collection on my desk.

Tuesday, Day 3

- Tending to my house plants, loving all their shades of green and marveling at the growth of new leaves.

- Feeling sweat pop and drip on my skin while I'm exercising.

- Smelling, visually appreciating and savoring my food that I prepare exactly as I desire.

- Driving my car in luxurious comfort and safety with music and sunshine pouring through the moonroof while loving the freedom to go anywhere I want, whenever I want.

- Watering the big pots of pink flowers on my porch and lawn while admiring how they and my rose bushes are bursting with red and pink blooms.

- Dwelling in my imagination to experience decadent visions and new levels of GoddessLife that I intend to manifest in my physical reality.

- Practicing the overwhelming feeling of gratitude by saying out loud, "Thank you, God!" and thinking about everything I'm thankful for.

Biss looks at all of you. "This is not frivolous. It's self-care! So let's talk about how to create an environment that intensifies your daily GoddessPleasure. It should be all about *you*. Not what's trending. Not what your parents or your partner/spouse/lover/bestie prefers. What delights *you?* If you live with other people and don't have the freedom to redecorate, then create your own private space. Create your GoddessSpace. Give it a fun name, like Zeusse's Zen Lounge or Andi's Attic or Bianca's Bayview Book Nook or Celeste's Sanctuary. Transform a closet, an attic or basement space, a bedroom if you're an empty nester, a shed, a camper. Be creative!"

Jade raises her hand. "I have a swing in my living room. It's like carved wood, as big as a twin bed, and has like a canopy over it. I put plants and little lights all around it. I go there to write songs or sometimes to just veg out."

"That's a great example," Biss says. "Think about how you can enhance every room of your home in ways that delight your eyes, ears, nose, skin and mind."

Kiki raises her hand. "When I get my own place, I want a sex room."

"Fun!" Biss exclaims. "More and more people are creating a sex room in their homes."

"What in the world is a sex room?" Delaney asks.

"It's a room designated for Pleasure," Biss says. "And it's a trend, as singles, couples and polyamorous people are hiring experts to design a room that caters to their wildest desires. I highly recommend watching the Netflix series, *How to Build a Sex Room*. It shows everyday people who want to make their sex lives blaze in a decadent space in their homes. Every episode will open your mind to new ideas while destigmatizing the human need for sexual exploration."

Biss smiles. "Let's take five minutes and write what you can do every day to enjoy micro-moments of sensual Pleasure in your home, workspace, car, cottage and any other place where you spend time."

_____

_____

_____

_____

Tuesday, Day 3

After five minutes of writing, Biss says, "Now before we dive into Sexual Pleasure, I want to talk about how you can use your sex energy to launch into your GoddessGenius Zone and experience creativity and focus as never before."

"Sex Transmutation" appears on the screen. Biss looks up. "Does anyone know what this means?"

The tent is silent.

"I didn't either," she says, "when I read *Think and Grow Rich* by Napoleon Hill. He has a whole chapter on this. But once I figured it out and tried it, I entered an era where my GoddessGenius Zone was blazing with creativity and productivity. It was nothing short of magic."

Andi asks, "So what is it?"

"It means channeling your sex energy into creativity," Biss says. "Sex energy is the most powerful energy in our bodies; its primary purpose is to create human life. Our energy centers that correspond to sex energy, sensuality and creativity are our root and sacral chakras, which are located around our sex organs, including our wombs, where human life can begin. So, when you channel that sensual and sexual energy into creating something—like starting a business, writing a book, or painting a portrait—you're tapping into supernatural fuel."

The screen above Biss shows the silhouette of a woman. Sparkling gold energy surges up from between her legs, through her body, into her brain, where it explodes around her head like a starburst.

"Sex transmutation has helped me write my *Husbands, Inc.* trilogy and so many other books," Biss says. "It's powerful because, when you abstain from sex—"

"What?!" Kiki exclaims.

"I knew there was a catch," Andi quips.

"Can't you be creative and have sex, too?" Sunshine asks.

Welcome to The Biss Tribe

"Of course you can," Biss says. "This concept is all about energy and priorities. Several of you have said you want to focus your energy on yourself and your businesses, as opposed to romance and/or hook-ups. That's because the activities around sex and the act itself can profoundly deplete our energy. And even though sex is one of life's greatest gifts, becoming aware of how draining it can be will help you make the best choices as you build your empires. Take it or leave it, but just hear me out."

Kiki crosses her arms. Celeste shakes her head.

"What if you could channel your sex energy to create a million-dollar business plan or some entrepreneurial innovation?" Biss asks. "Rather than allowing the energy to leave the body through a sexual release, what if you channeled it up to your mind and through your chakra system to connect with the infinite power of Source?"

Jade raises her hand. "I'm doing that. I have no sex right now, and I've been writing songs in my genius zone, for sure."

Biss nods. "Sex transmutation isn't all about sex. It's also about the energy of pursuing, engaging and resting after. Years ago, I reached a point where I awakened to the infuriating reality that romantic relationships were draining my energy and derailing my dreams."

Biss shakes her head. "Not tryin' to be Debbie Downer, because I love men and romance and the thrills that it brings. But then I thought about the shopping, cleaning, getting ready to see him, spending time with him, cleaning up, and resting because we stayed up late. And if a relationship was causing me anxiety, anger or worse, that was an infuriating distraction from writing my books. I hated it! I couldn't concentrate and I was exhausted."

Sunshine lights up. "Now I get it. That's the same for me. And as soon as I end the relationship, I can focus really well again."

"Thank you, Sunshine," Biss says.

Tuesday, Day 3

"Biss, now that you have a partner," Zeusse says, "do you still practice sex transmutation?"

"I have a partner who enhances everything I do," Biss says. "We have a routine where he honors my need for eight solid hours of sleep every night, and my need for solitude during long hours when I'm writing. So I don't have to abstain."

"That's what's up," Zeusse says. "To find your boo who vibes with you like that."

Know Your Own Body First

Sensuous and beautiful watercolor paintings of nude women appear on the screen.

"Before you can experience the ultimate Pleasure," Biss says, "it's imperative to **know your own body**. What your female parts look like, how you like to stimulate yourself, and the best way to bring yourself to orgasm. This will enhance your experience with a partner or partners, because you'll know what you like, and have the courage to express it. And if you're with someone who disregards that, or does not provide a safe space for you to express what you want, they are not the person for you! Run!"

Sunshine shakes her head. "That's been me too many times. I'd rather be alone until I find my husband."

Bianca raises her hand. "My fear issues make it really hard to speak up, because I've had guys get really angry and storm out of the bedroom when I've asked for what I want. They took it as an insult."

Biss nods. "I've been there, too, and there's always the safety factor when you're alone with a man in the nude. The best case scenario is to talk about things before you're in a vulnerable position, say, while taking a walk together in public. See how they react, and decide accordingly whether you'll proceed to the bedroom."

"I like that," Jade says.

"If this makes you uncomfortable and you feel, *Oh I was taught that was just not right for girls or women, or it's sinful, or that's only for my man or my husband to take however he wants—*"

Biss shakes her head and playfully says, "*Screech! Screech* to a halt! It's *your* body. And it's your birthright to know it, understand it, and enjoy it. This is a no judgment zone. All I care about is that you maximize your own Pleasure, and sometimes the only thing that's standing in the way of you doing that is a mindset shift by lifting off oppressive beliefs."

Women's Pleasure Centers 101

The screen above Biss says, "The Anatomy of GoddessPleasure."

"Hopefully this is redundant for all of you," she says. " But if not, it's imperative that you understand your own anatomy to fully experience Pleasure by yourself. Plus, if *you* don't understand it, how can you expect your lover to navigate your body parts to Pleasure you at maximum capacity?"

The screen shows video animation of a baby in the womb, with images corresponding to what she's saying.

"We're born with a little bubble of flesh called the clitoris, also known as a clit," she says. "In the womb, it forms from the same protrusion of flesh that becomes a penis. Lucky for girls, all 10,281 nerve endings[2] are concentrated in this one spot. That's why it's so sensitive to touch."

The screen shows video animation of a woman's external sex organs, highlighted by purple flashing arrows as Biss describes them, starting with the clitoris.

"This is the major Pleasure center for most women, along with the G-spot inside the vagina. These are the labia, the lips."

Tuesday, Day 3

Biss looks out at you and the women. "When I took women's studies classes in college, I learned that many women have never used a mirror to look between their legs. So, if that's you, no shame, but please do this with the mirror and light you'll find in your private tent."

The tent fills with in a chorus of: "I've never done that," and "Oh my God, how embarrassing."

Marla says to Sammie, "Remember how Jenna got va-jay-jay lip surgery because her boyfriend said they were too big? Horrible."

Sammie twists her face and says, "Never would I *ever!*"

They focus back on Biss, who says, "Now, look at this. Between the labia is the clitoris. Just as arousal causes blood to flow into the penis and it becomes erect, arousal also causes blood to flow into the clitoris, and it swells while the vagina naturally lubricates and feels wet. The biological reason for this is for a penis to easily enter to create a pregnancy."

Biss aims the purple dot on a little hole at the tip of the clitoris.

"The clitoris is also like a hood over the urethra, where your pee comes out, from the urethra, which connects to your bladder." She aims at the vagina. "Here's where menstrual blood and babies come out. And where a penis or fingers or a dildo go in for sexual Pleasure. The vagina leads up to a firm circle of tissue called the cervix, which is the entrance to the uterus, where babies grow."

The women are silent and still.

"This is super embarrassing," Marla says. "Nobody has ever explained this to me."

"I'm glad to be the first." Biss pauses. "I can feel how uncomfortable some of you are with this. That's exactly why we need to talk about it, meditate on it, and take action to normalize this information and conversation."

One woman says, "My mom didn't tell me anything. She didn't even show me what to do when I got my period. She just handed me a box of tampons and pads and said, 'Use these.' And take Tylenol for cramps."

Several women echo similar comments.

"It's really important to get comfortable with your body and your own genitalia," Biss says. "First, as a matter of health, you need to know what looks and feels normal, so if anything changes, you can get it checked out. Second, because it's your body, and it can bring you amazing Pleasure."

Orgasms!

Sexy hip hop music blasts and the dancers bust back onto the stage, immediately shifting the energy from embarrassed and awkward to fun and energetic as many women snap their fingers and shimmy on their sofas.

"It's time for GoddessPleasure!" Biss shouts as the dancers circle her. "We're here to unleash it—big, loud and bodaciously!"

The women cheer.

"So now let's talk about the bliss of orgasms," Biss says. "Did you know they have a long list of health benefits for your brain and body? And they can help your GoddessVoice and GoddessVision attune to the universal field of knowledge to receive downloads that help you build your empire?"

Celeste laughs. "I am all ears! Can't wait to hear *this!*"

Sunshine raises her hand to her face as if to shield it from the sun. "Oh my God, this is so embarrassing!"

Whispers of, "I know, right!" and "Eeek!" ripple from the women.

The screen shows an animated starburst of light radiating from a woman's blissful face as she lounges on a bed.

"First, orgasms make you glow," Biss says. "Your skin becomes more clear and radiant, your eyes sparkle and your energy increases. Your confidence boosts, because you realize, *I made my*

Tuesday, Day 3

body do that. At the same time, orgasms cause chemical reactions in your body that make you glow!"

Biss flashes a huge smile. "A few years ago, I was in a restaurant and bumped into a girlfriend who said, 'Biss, you're just glowing! You look like a goddess. What's your secret?' She really said that, and I hadn't event started my Goddess programs. So I just smiled and whispered, 'Amazing orgasms.' She looked shocked and envious, but the next time I saw her, she was radiant! She winked at me, flashed a giant smile, and said, 'You inspired me.'"

On stage, a new dancer appears, beating a drum while other dancers surround Biss, creating a pulsating movement, up and down, with their arms and backs moving in sensuous unison.

"My mission is for all of you to have that moment," Biss says, "where someone looks at you and says, 'What's your secret?' And you say, 'I activated my GoddessPleasure in The Biss Tribe.' Sound good?"

Marla shouts, "Hell yeah, bitches!"

"Best news ever!" Jade yells.

"Can't do it soon enough," Andi calls into the women's loud cheering. "Scares the shit outta me, but it's now or never, man."

Biss beams up at you and the women. "So let's do this!"

She steps in front of the dancers—a tangle of writhing limbs and sparkling costumes.

"Here are more benefits of orgasm beyond the Pleasure of the moment," she exclaims. "Your mood improves, thanks to a release of feel-good hormones that include oxytocin. This diminishes stress—along with your chances of stress-induced illness. In fact, scientific research shows that oxytocin lowers levels of cortisol, the stress hormone that can cause health catastrophes, including heart attacks and strokes. Imagine, orgasms can actually save your life by improving the chemical balances in your body."

"I had no idea," Delaney says in amazement.

Welcome to The Biss Tribe

"And look at all these benefits!" Words stream across the screen as Biss talks:

"Orgasms: help you live longer... improve your immunity... relieve pain... reduce anxiety... boost your self-esteem... energize you... relax you... improve your body image... help you bond with your partner... help you sleep... make you smile... feel amazing... improve your mental focus... and celebrate the beautiful gifts that we're born with in our amazing bodies!"[3]

Biss has an excited expression as she scans the rows of women. "Tonight in your private tents, you'll find a special chair with an attached light and mirror that will enable you to look at your genitalia. You'll also find a toybox with a variety of stimulating devices. And your Concierge will be available to assist you to explain how the toys work, and how to use them. They will respect your boundaries. And they will go as far as you'd like, with safety being the top priority. You can do this with your current Concierge, or you can request a male, female or nonbinary Concierge. And if you prefer to be alone, that's fine as well."

Jade raises her tattooed arm. "I definitely want help."

The screen shows a variety of colorful sex toys. "In your personal toybox," Biss says, "you'll find vibrators, dildos and amazing biotech devices that mimic human touch and tongues."

Zeusse lets out a low laugh. "That's what's up!"

"Holy shit!" Andi looks shocked. "What *are* all those things!?"

Video on the screen shows the toys buzzing and moving and rotating.

"These are some of the greatest inventions ever!" Biss looks up at the screen. "Experiment with them. Discover what you like most. In your tent, use the plush lounge chair with the angled mirror and light to see what you're doing. Explore your erogenous zones. Play and be open to new experiences."

Tuesday, Day 3

Several women shift nervously. "This is way out of my comfort zone," a woman says.

"Good!" Biss smiles. "That's the point. I'm here to argue that your comfort zone is a trap that keeps you stuck. Apply that to every area of your life. Especially when it comes to Pleasure."

Andi lets out a groan. "Talk about taboo, man. I got caught playing with myself in the bathtub as a kid, and my Gramma spanked the living shit outta me. Then she said, 'You bad girl! You remember this! Anything between a girl's legs is the devil's workshop, unless she's married and letting her husband do his business to make a baby.'"

Delaney shakes her head. "I was brainwashed with the same garbage, and unfortunately, it's robbed me of too much Pleasure over my lifetime."

Sammie looks disgusted. "Don't even get me started about slut shaming on social media. They want us to look and act sexy, but the minute they don't like something, or you break up, these ruthless dudes will put AI porn with your face all over social media."

"Or pictures and vids you shared with them," Marla adds. "Revenge porn is a thing. It's horrible!"

Biss shakes her head. "That's a reality of this world, sadly. You decide how to navigate that, and weigh the consequences of staying in fear and letting life pass you by without fully liberating your sexuality, *or* living out loud and not giving half a flying fuck what anyone thinks."

Sunshine says softly, "That fear is paralyzing. I never want to be called a ho and I hate so much that we as women have to consider our safety, health and reputation before we can just be free to do everything you're saying. All while guys do everything so freely and easily, and get celebrated for it!"

Biss nods. "That's all real talk, my Goddesses. And that's why you're here. To escape that shame and secrecy and fear around

Welcome to The Biss Tribe

sex. Pleasure is our birthright! It's ours for the taking! That's why I'm giving you all permission to give *yourself* permission to feel comfortable and emboldened to enjoy the Pleasures of your own body!"

Sammie and many women are quiet, while others cheer.

The image of Archangel Raphael appears on the screen. "My dear Goddesses! Please repeat the healing meditation at home until every last speck of shame, fear and guilt is out of your system. You'll leave the retreat with an audio recording that will guide you through it."

Jade sighs. "I thought I was pretty liberated, but this conversation is giving me the ick."

"Same!" Marla and Sammie say in unison as many women nod.

Biss shakes her head. "Your reactions make me all the more motivated to teach this. You deserve Pleasure! On your terms! And once you have your GoddessPleasure Awakening, with or without a partner, you'll never be the same. It will ignite confidence and courage inside you that you have to feel to believe. That's where I live and love every damn day, and I've never been happier. I want that for *you!*"

The screen shows video of several couples holding hands and cuddling.

"I'm here to help you set a new standard on sexual satisfaction," Biss says. "Activating your GoddessPleasure means you demand of yourself and your lover or lovers that you always enjoy Pleasure to the max. As I said, Pleasure is the portal to your Power, because it puts you in tune with your body, shatters taboos and elevates you to the highest frequency vibration of joy, love and peace that opens a supernatural gateway into another dimension where the electric current of the universe activates your GoddessPleasure and Power."

The music booms and the dancers reappear, pulsing in formation around Biss. She casts a sultry glance at them, then smiles.

Tuesday, Day 3

"Thanks to Dream Lover," Biss says, "I want extraordinary Pleasure or nothing at all. If my lover can't make my skin feel like it's shimmering with diamonds from the top of my head to my curling toes, then that's a deal breaker. I believe that great, uninhibited, intense sex is imperative for the success of a romantic relationship, especially if it's allegedly going to be exclusive—and that's a whole different conversation for another day."

The dancers pair off as couples, staring intensely into each other's eyes and doing sensuous dances in perfect synchronicity with each other.

"If this were easy," Biss says, "you wouldn't be here. So, here are a few tips for ensuring satisfaction when you're with a partner. First, if you feel that your partner is unwilling to revive the passion, affection and communication with you, then take time alone and contemplate whether you really want to stay in the relationship, even if it's a long-term marriage."

A few women exhale with exasperation.

"If you feel emotionally malnourished," Biss says, "and I've been there and it's horrible, feeling lonely in the same bed with—but disconnected from—the person who's supposed to love you, then that's a terrible way to spend the rest of your life. You have to decide if you want to stay. You deserve to feel fulfilled with your partner."

You listen as the women are still and silent.

"Now, if you're in a relationship or situationship worth keeping," Biss says, "you have to tell them what you want. If you like to be touched a certain way—or not—then describe or demonstrate your preferences. If your person bullishly disregards what you request and thinks they know a better way—but they don't, that shows their insensitive personality and potential incompatibility in a relationship."

"That was my X," Sunshine says.

"Mine, too," Biss says. "Emphasis on X. Likewise, if you love toys, but your person 'prohibits' toys, that's a deal-breaker. The bedroom is a microcosm for the rest of the relationship, and if they're unwilling to make you happy there, that reflects other issues. It's complicated, and there's much more to life than sex. But if they're not pleasing you, you can take matters into your own hands, literally."

"Communication" appears on the screen with video of a couple sitting and talking on a sofa.

"Unless your partner is psychic and can read your mind," Biss says, "you have to tell them what you like and want. This takes courage, and should be expressed in a way that doesn't sound like criticism. So my first tip is to know what you want, and write out a script in your journal of how to say it. You can practice in the mirror or rehearse with a friend who can provide potential responses that your partner might have."

"Wow, I love that idea," Jade says.

"You can also tell your partner what you like about their lovemaking skills, and say, 'I'd really love it if you can be more gentle, or rougher, or let's try new positions or do it in the bathtub.' A helpful exercise is to think through how you would respond if your lover asked you to perform oral sex with a different technique. Would you feel criticized? Your ability to express yourself is rooted in two things: your own confidence and comfort with your Pleasure, and the vibe with your partner, and whether you feel safe to express yourself and ask for what you want."

In the front row, Phyllis raises her hand. "What if you're in a long-term marriage and you've never had the guts to speak up and you've always just let him do his thing without asking for what you want?"

"That can be tricky," Biss says, "because the partner may feel defensive or suspicious that you've been unfaithful and learned new things that you want to bring home to them."

Sunshine groans. "I hated it when my X did that; I always knew he'd been with someone else when he wanted to try some new wild position."

Biss nods, then looks at Phyllis. "I highly recommend that you work with a trusted sex therapist who provides a safe space where you and your partner can talk openly and honestly about unmet needs in the bedroom. You can broach the subject by watching a series like *Couples Therapy*, then ease into the idea of doing that yourselves."

"That scares the shit outta me," Phyllis says. "My girlfriend got her ass beat when she asked her husband to last longer so she could cum."

Biss scowls. "I'm so sorry to hear that."

"And you talk about self-Pleasure," Phyllis says, "but another friend got smacked when her boyfriend walked in on her playing with herself. He said, 'That's mine! And only I get to decide when you get some sex.'"

Many women groan with disgust.

"Possessive and violent behaviors like those indicate much bigger problems in the relationship," Biss says, "that are all too common. So please navigate this with safety first. And any woman who's in an unsafe relationship, should create a safe, solid strategy to escape."

"What a buzz kill, man," Andi says.

"For sure," Jade adds.

"Very sobering," Delaney says.

"But reality," Biss says. "Because women are viewed as property and our sexuality is perceived as something that men feel entitled to control. I'm not a sex therapist or a psychologist. But I strongly recommend that one, you navigate your relationships in a way that keeps you safe. Two, you seriously consider leaving any relationship that stifles you in ways that we just discussed. And three, that you carefully vet future partners to determine their mindset when it comes to your sexual freedom."

Phyllis raises her hand. "So many women are trapped in relationships and marriages when they have kids and no money. They stay because they have nowhere else to go. Even my affluent friends, they stay in marriages they hate because it would be so expensive and disruptive to their lifestyle and social life and professional status together."

Biss has a blank expression. "That's their choice. And being here is *your* choice. Learning how to activate your Power, Pleasure, Prosperity, Protection and Peace, liberates you to build your own empire that provides the freedom to live and love as you truly desire."

"Amen!" Celeste exclaims as Zeusse says, "That's what's up!" Marla and Sammie say, "Hell yeah, bitches!" And other women cheer.

Explore & Enjoy Self-Pleasure!

The screen shows a woman alone, lounging in a sensuous position.

"Let's talk about self-Pleasure," Biss says. "I use that term instead of 'masturbation,' which sounds so clinical and not fun. Self-Pleasure should be a major part of every woman's daily self-care routine."

Jade looks perplexed. "Why are we taught that something that's good for us is a sin? That's so freaking stupid!"

"One hundred percent," Zeusse says. "It's puritanical."

Tuesday, Day 3

"I encourage you to indulge in self-Pleasure as frequently as possible," Biss says, "at least several times each week. This is all about you. Nobody else. Whether you're married or living with a mate or dating someone, you have the right to Pleasure yourself in the privacy of your home. No one has to know."

The dancers shimmy around Biss, then synchronize in wave motions toward you and the women.

"And again, if you feel you need permission to embrace your sexuality," Biss says, "I'm giving it to you now. So, more on devices that can enhance your self-Pleasure."

The screen shows another array of vibrators, dildos, and objects that elicit whispers of, "What's that!?"

Biss laughs. "Toys will rock your world! You can buy stimulators of all types, and sex toys are high-tech now. You can even buy something that simulates the suction sensations of someone performing oral sex on you. You can use battery-powered vibrators that stimulate your clit, and even plug-in ones, like Kiki and Celeste mentioned earlier."

A colorful assortment of things that look like microphones appears on the screen.

"You can also get plug-in 'wands' that vibrate at 9,000 RPMs and will send you into orgasmic shudders that you have to experience to believe," Biss says. "Pair that with a dildo for vaginal stimulation, and your mind will be blown!"

Excited whispers ripple through the tent.

"When you return for your Biss Tribe Intensive here at the Pleasure Tent, we'll have demonstrations and vendors so you can purchase whatever you want. You'll also get to participate in private and group sessions with sex therapists who will open your minds and Pleasure centers in amazing ways."

Biss points to more toys flashing across the screen.

"Of course, every woman is different," she says. "If you don't like penetration, then skip it. If you're super sensitive and need low-voltage stimulation, find that. If you love penetration, you can find a dildo that's the perfect size for you. And if your partner is female, she can strap on and blow your mind. Or your man can use it to supplement the real deal."

A woman's butt with a light glowing between her cheeks appears on the screen. "If you like anal penetration, you can get butt plugs that vibrate, creating a triple-whammy experience if you also use a dildo for vaginal stimulation and a vibrator on your clit."

Bianca raises her hand. "I must have been living in a cave. I've never heard of any of this. Where do you buy this stuff?"

"In a lingerie shop, an adult toy store, or online," Biss says. "You can watch videos made by bold women who do product reviews for sex toys. It's also fun to visit a sex toy store and explore. Don't be embarrassed! The people who work there are excited to help you find exactly what you want, and the other shoppers are doing the same thing. While you're at it, these stores also make it easy to buy sexy fashions for the boudoir—lingerie, bras, panties, body stockings, crotchless things, costumes, and even shoes and boots. Mostly, have fun!"

Let's Close the Orgasm Gap

Words stream across the screen above Biss:

> **Orgasm:** The rapid pleasurable release of neuromuscular tensions at the height of sexual arousal... usually accompanied by the ejaculation of semen in the male and by vaginal contractions in the female.[4]

Tuesday, Day 3

Biss reads the words, then an animated video shows a penis squirting inside a vagina, followed by a stream of sperm swimming up into the upside-down triangle, into a fallopian tube, where one sperm pierces the surface of a plump egg, which floats into the uterus, and a baby starts to grow.

"Now let's talk about biology for a minute," Biss says. "The function for orgasm in men is to spray sperm into the vagina, so the sperm can swim up through the cervix, into the uterus and fallopian tubes, and fertilize an egg to create a baby, which keeps the human race going."

Biss looks annoyed. "Unfortunately, throughout history, this act has been all about the man's pleasure, while women's orgasms have been denied, ignored, discounted and deemed irrelevant."

The screen shows video of a couple in bed. The man is super happy, lounging and grinning, while the woman is lying on her side with her back to him. She looks sad and mad.

"Who's ever been in this position?" Biss asks.

A chorus of "me!" erupts.

"We have to close the orgasm gap!" Biss exclaims.

"What's that?" Celeste asks.

Biss answers: "It's like the Gender Pay Gap, where women earn 84 cents for every dollar a man makes, and the numbers are more dismal for women of color, according to the U.S. Department of Labor."[5]

Biss shakes her head. "Well, there's a gap in the bedroom, too. Men orgasm about 85% of the time, but heterosexual women only orgasm 64% of the time, according to a study by researchers at the Kinsey Institute for Research in Sex, Gender, and Reproduction at Indiana University."[6]

Numbers flash on the screen as Biss says, "The study also showed that lesbian women orgasm more with a partner, nearly

75% of the time. No surprise. If you know how to Pleasure yourself, you know what another woman would like."

Zeusse smiles. "That's what's up. I make sure my females *all* have their GoddessPleasure Awakening with me."

Andi casts an envious glance at Zeusse.

Jade smiles, too. "I always orgasm with women, but with guys, not so much. They just get theirs and it's over. Hate that. So much!"

Celeste shakes her head. "I had to teach my husband what to do. Happy wife, happy life. Especially in the bedroom."

"So how do we close the orgasm gap?" Marla asks.

"By first becoming aware of it," Biss says. "Then by doing everything here that you're learning to activate your GoddessPleasure. Third, by helping other women shatter the stigma around their sexuality."

Words pop onto the screen: anal... cervical... nipple... exercise... sleep... multiple... clitoral... vagina... g-spot.

"We'll dive deep into the history of women's orgasms when you return here to The Pleasure Tent for your Intensive," Biss says. "For now, let's talk about three main types of orgasms."

The screen shows animation of a starburst exploding from a woman's pelvis.

"First is **Clitoral**," Biss says, "achieved by stimulating the clitoris with fingers, a mouth and/or toys. Next is **Vaginal**. With the right ferocity, duration and stroke, your partner who knows how to work a penis, dildo and/or fingers—can give you vaginal orgasms. So can you, by yourself, with a dildo. And the third main type of orgasm is the **Blended Orgasm** or what I call the **Double Whammy**."

The starburst on the woman on the screen glows brighter and bigger, consuming her entire being.

"Clitoral and vaginal stimulation at the same time can give you *ridiculous* orgasms," Biss says. "Your homework tonight is to explore what works best for you, by yourself. Then you can share that with your partner or partners when you get home."

Sammie gasps. "Not me for a whole year! But in the past, when I wanted to tell a guy how to do me, I'd get so scared, I couldn't even make a sentence. I thought he'd take it as an insult to his skills."

"He would!" Sunshine says. "I tried that, and it didn't go well. Especially with a narcissist who thinks he knows everything and does everything the best."

Bianca nods. "My ex-husband told me he didn't want me to use any toys that could make me feel better than he did. He also thought I couldn't enjoy sex after the accident, even though I told him I can still orgasm, thankfully."

Kiki says, "One dude told me if I want toys, it means he's not enough. He wasn't!"

"Girlfriend," Celeste says, "your lover should make it his top priority to please you just the way you want. That's a real man. Stop messin' with boys."

"Fuck boys," Sammie quips. "I'm so done with those mother fuckers. Literally."

Delaney shakes her head. "Unfortunately, boys like that come in all ages. I finally learned to speak up for what I want and never settle for less than that. But it didn't happen for many years. So please, ladies," she says, looking at you and all the women, "don't let that be you."

"Thank you for that, Delaney," Biss says.

Marla sinks into her chair. "This is so embarrassing."

"Why is it embarrassing?" Biss asks.

"I don't know," she says, "I just feel hot and prickly. Even though this is exactly what I came here to overcome. I mean, I've never even had an orgasm."

Sammie beams. "Tonight might be the night, when you get in there with all those toys."

"Orgasmic Visualization & Creation" streams across the screen above Biss, followed by the definition, which she reads:

"Orgasmic Visualization means envisioning what you want in vivid detail during Pleasure and while orgasming, as a way to manifest your desires into physical reality."

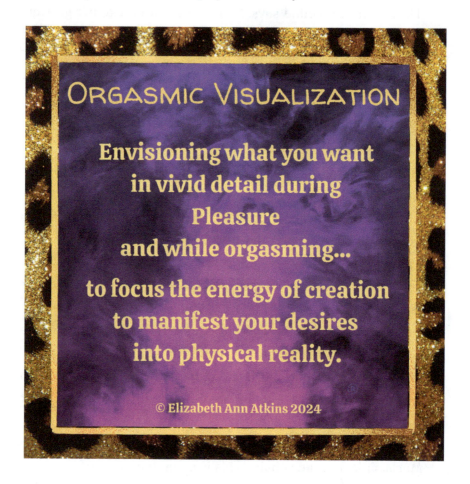

"Whoah," Andi says. "Let me wrap my brain around that one."

"I don't get it," Jade says.

"How are you supposed to concentrate on something while you're trying to get off?" Kiki asks.

Tuesday, Day 3

"Why would we want to be distracted during sex to do that?" Sunshine asks.

"Because this really works!" Biss says. "When you combine the power of your mind to visualize what you want, and infuse it with the powerful energy of creation that explodes during orgasm, you're harnessing that energy to help you manifest what you want."

"I don't think I could concentrate," Andi says. "It's too overwhelming."

Biss nods. "It takes practice to concentrate on something in the heat of the moment. It also requires belief that it will work, along with action to help make it happen. But during that explosive moment when you energize your vision with your body's luscious, life-creating energy, it activates something inside you and in the universe to make it happen."

Delaney asks, "Can you do this with a partner if you both focus on the same goal while you're making love? Seems like it would double the manifestation power."

"Exactly!" Biss says. "That takes us into tantric sex, where two people enjoy an extraordinary union of mind, body and soul."

The screen shows animated video of a nude couple facing each other as the woman straddles the man's lap. He's sitting with his legs crossed and her legs are wrapped around him. They're staring into each other's eyes, arms embracing each other, and breathing each other's breath as colorful waves of light radiate outward from them.

"That's beautiful," Sunshine says longingly. "I want my husband to be open to doing things like that with me. Like next-level lovemaking."

"Yes," Biss says. "Has anyone ever tried orgasmic visualization and creation?"

"Never heard of it!" Phyllis says. "So how do you do it?"

"First, set the intention," Biss says. "Decide what you want to focus on. Then, as you engage in self-Pleasure or sex with your partner, enjoy the experience, but also bring your thoughts back to envisioning what you want. Picture it vividly in your mind as an image or even filmstrip, as if you've already manifest it in physical reality. At the same time, you can give thanks to Spirit and ask Spirit to reveal anything you need to know about how to make it happen."

"Sounds like erotic meditation," Kiki says.

"Good one, Kiki," Biss says. "That's exactly it. Because sometimes during orgasm, you can receive a vision or a message from Spirit. It's really psychedelic."

"How though?" Sunshine asks.

"Just be open to listening and seeing any messages that Spirit wants to deliver while you're in the supernatural portal of sexual bliss."

The screen says, "La Petite Mort."

"Does anyone know what this means?" Biss asks.

"That's French for 'the little death,'" Sammie says, "but what's that got to do with Pleasure?"

"La Petite Mort is the term French people use to describe an orgasm," Biss explains. "It's like a little death. And what happens when someone dies? Their soul goes into the heavenly realm, which is supernatural."

"I have chills," Sunshine says as several women exclaim, "Wow."

"So," Biss says, "this highlights the fact that orgasms ignite supernatural energy that you can use to manifest your GoddessLife."

Tuesday, Day 3

Sounding the Alarms in Your GoddessPleasure Mission Control Center

Animated video of a woman flying a glass airplane appears on the screen.

"This may be your most dangerous flight," Biss says. "Just like we talked yesterday about friends, family and society trying to hijack your personal Mission Control Tower, to dictate how you can or cannot navigate the flight patterns of your GoddessLife, this will be especially treacherous when it comes to Pleasure."

On the video, buttons on the airplane's control panel start flashing red and beeping and sounding alarms.

"You better believe," Biss says, "you will hear all kinds of noise from the 'powers that be' who want you to follow their flight pattern in the Good Girl Zone."

"Rebel bitches, unite!" Marla yells. Several women laugh.

"So," Biss says, "you can choose to fly in secret. You can choose to fly far away from the critical eyes of your family, friends, colleagues, faith community and neighbors... by either doing things discreetly, or by moving to a new town."

"That's why I'm opening my beachfront art studio in Provincetown," Andi says. "Lots of rainbow flags flying there, so I can live out loud and proud. Finally."

Kiki raises a hand. "I've met lots of people in the Lifestyle. That's what you call people who are swingers. At one party, I was shocked to see prominent lawyers, doctors and executives. They live a wild life behind closed doors, but in public, they're mega respected and nobody knows what wild freaks they are. In the Lifestyle, your kinks stay secret."

Sunshine looks baffled. "Why have I never heard of any of this?"

"Exactly what I just said," Kiki adds. "It's easy to find if you're looking for it. On membership websites, on social media, and at events."

"Not for me," Sunshine says.

"Me either," Celeste adds. "But it's interesting."

"You," Biss says, "have the Power to decide how you'll fly your symbolic airplane in your GodddessLife. You can choose to flaunt your newfound sexual liberation by putting on a sky show with dramatic flight patterns that scroll fluffy white messages in the sky with smoke from your plane. Or you can choose to fly under the radar, behind cover of darkness or shrouded in mysterious clouds, for discreet indulgence. For example, if you discover that you prefer a non-monogamous lovestyle, and you want to experience swingers parties and even nudist resorts and sex cruises, you can do this privately. You don't have to ask anyone's permission."

The screen shows video of a giant pool party with people laughing, drinking and dancing.

"Just always put safety first and find a trusted partner and/or group of like-minded people, and enjoy." Biss smiles. "I once asked a friend who has a prominent career, 'What if you go to one of those sex clubs and see someone who knows you?' And my friend said, 'I'm seeing them there, too!'"

The video screen shows people talking over drinks at the pool party. "Just like Kiki said, my friend told me that people in the Lifestyle practice a code of conduct that emphasizes confidentiality. They communicate openly and honestly and set boundaries. So if this interests you, watch videos online about people who are exploring nontraditional ways of living and loving, and decide if it's for you."

"It's not!" Andi says. "I want old fashioned one-on-one."

"Not me," Jade says. "I want to learn more. Traditional is not my thing."

Biss nods. "Expanding your knowledge about options is especially important if you don't want to conform to the hetero-monogamous template that society provides as the acceptable norm. A Goddess has the Power to decide who she is, what she wants, how she'll live and love, and who gets the honor and privilege of sharing time and attention with her. Remember that!"

The music blasts as the dancers explode around Biss in a shimmer of sparkly costumes and sensuous movement.

"My Goddesses!" Biss exclaims. "This concludes our time here in The Pleasure Tent, until you return for your Pleasure Intensive in a few months. For now, everybody say, 'Pleasure is the portal to my GoddessPower! I deserve Pleasure every day!'"

You and the women repeat that with Biss as the dancers provide a dizzying, dazzling performance that ends with them dancing up the center and side steps, rousing many women to stand and dance with them.

"Ladies," Esmerelda announces, "after a restroom break, please follow me onto the Pleasure Trail for a refreshing walk with Mother Nature."

Take a Refreshing Walk on the Pleasure Trail

A short time later, you and all the women are walking outdoors on a picturesque trail amidst flowers, trees, rocks and groves with swing chairs where you're welcome to sit, journal, talk and meditate. The Concierges and security guards follow as Esmerelda sets a brisk pace; Bianca is in her power chair, which rides smoothly over the hard dirt trail.

"Ladies," Esmerelda says, leading you into a tree- and flower-shaded clearing beside a trickling stream. "Please spread out and let's stretch."

She leads you and all the women through a series of stretches.

"This feels amazing," Marla says.

"I'm stretching muscles I didn't know I had," Jade adds.

"Can't wait to see what's for dinner," another woman quips.

"Stay in the moment," Sunshine says, raising her arms to the sky. "Right now is a gift. That's why it's called the present."

Welcome to Your Personal GoddessPleasure Tent

After the walk, Concierge Jami leads you to your private tent, which is nestled amidst lush landscaping and 30 tents behind the large one where you spent the day. The other women are entering their tents, which are round and covered in jewel-tone shades of fabric: emerald-green, cobalt blue, electric purple, gold and turquoise. Tassels, flags and sparkly drapes adorn each tent; Moroccan-style lanterns flank the draped entrances.

As you enter your tent, it feels spacious and dreamy, with huge swaths of satin swooping from the center ceiling pole to the tops of the walls. Hanging Moroccan-style lanterns cast colorful, stencil-like patterns on the low, loungey sofa, chairs and table, as well as the bed. It's round and draped with tulle that cascades down from a bed crown and shrouds a velvet bedspread and plush pillows.

Your favorite aromatherapy scents waft through the tent as Concierge Jami leads you to the luxurious bathroom. It has a sunken bathtub, a pretty assortment of soaps and bubble bath accessories, a huge mirror and vanity that holds vases of live orchids, and thick towels.

Jami opens the doors to a walk-in closet and says, "Here you'll find customized clothing for the GoddessFeast, and for sleeping and wearing on tomorrow's bus trip up to The GoddessTreasure Cave." They point to clothing on hangers. "The attire for this

Tuesday, Day 3

evening is a bathing suit as the foundation, with your selection of coverings that look festive and most importantly are very comfortable."

"Why the bathing suit?" you ask.

"So that you can, if you desire, sit in the hot springs and enjoy the relaxation and health benefits of the rich minerals in the water."

Concierge Jami opens a small door into a cozy little room that feels even more plush than the main space. You behold a chaise lounge-style chair with rectangular pillows to elevate your legs. A light and a mirror stand on silver poles beside it. And nearby is a large trunk covered in purple velvet and brass hardware. Concierge Jami opens it to reveal a colorful array of devices.

"Your toybox," Jami says. "Your assignment for this evening is self-discovery and Pleasure. I or another Concierge of your choosing will be available to explain and demonstrate how these devices work, and to provide any assistance you may need. We practice the utmost safety protocols and respect of your privacy and boundaries, and you are free to explore alone."

As you look into the toybox at the colorful shapes and sizes of each item, Concierge Jami says, "Also know that every device is safety-sealed and brand new in its original packaging."

Next, in the main room, they point to a mini bar with baskets of fruit, chocolates, wine, water, and pods for coffee, tea and hot chocolate. "You'll find more refreshments in this mini-refrigerator and you can make hot beverages with this single-serve coffee machine."

Concierge Jami steps toward the door. "I'll give you 30 minutes to freshen up and change clothes, and I will return to escort you to the GoddessFeast on the terrace."

The GoddessFeast on the Pleasure Tent Terrace

You arrive at The GoddessPleasure Tent Terrace along with the other women and their Concierges. You're amazed at how comfortable you feel in the bathing suit-based outfit that fits you perfectly and is your favorite style.

"I love this!" Marla says, striking a pose with Sammie in their matching, glittering pink bikini tops and flouncy ballerina-style skirts, as a string quartet plays sensuous music.

You marvel at all the variations of the women's outfits that reflect their personalities with elegance and varying degrees of modesty. At the foundation are strappy, bodycon-type bikinis or one-pieces made of opalescent, stretchy fabric. They are covered by skirts, blouses, dresses, flowy pants and tunics made of sheer, opalescent tulle, satin or linen.

Kiki wears a black bandeau covered by a dramatic, poufy sheer blouse tied at the waist with an ankle-length skirt that has high slits up the sides.

Celeste's one-piece has thick diagonal straps that accentuate her chest, framed by dark purple sheer jacket whose feathers flounce around her hips over wide-legged, pleated satin pants.

Andi and Zeusse wear white linen trousers and button-up shirts that open just enough to reveal a tank top underneath.

"I can't wait to get in the hot springs," Sunshine says, wearing a turquoise explosion of ruffles over a strappy bikini top.

Bianca's outfit is similar. She points to her turquoise hair and smiles, saying, "It's important for your clothes to match your hair and braces."

"You got style, sis!" Jade says, doing the GoddessGreeting with Bianca.

Tuesday, Day 3

"My outfit matches my tatts," Jade says, pointing to the goddesses and vines adorning her arms that match her emerald-green one-piece under a sleeveless, double-breasted satin dress coat whose buttons are rhinestone guitars.

"I'm loving the innovation of this fashion," Delaney adds, whose white one-piece peeks from the vee-neck of a long satin tunic dress. "And how we're all wearing our crystal jewelry." She touches her black tourmaline pendant and bracelets, that are identical to the ones that you and every woman are wearing.

"Look at this place!" Marla says with awe as the Concierges lead you onto the terrace that overlooks the vast valley below. Early evening sunshine casts a golden glow over a U-shaped table whose opening faces a small stage holding two purple throne chairs. They're framed by draping magenta satin suspended by a gold crown whose ornate pattern matches the wood around the velvet thrones. A Moroccan-style metal lantern hangs between the chairs over a small table where a vase bursts with colorful flowers.

Beyond the large dining table, steam rises from the oval-shaped pool that's fed by the hot springs. Surrounding the pool are boulders and raised circles of rocks that are unlit fire pits. Between the hot springs pool and the dining area, on a slightly elevated platform, DJ Panther is setting up her booth that overlooks a dance floor that's surrounded by Moroccan-lantern style string lights.

"Tonight will be so fun," Sammie says as you and the women take your seats at the table.

"I can't wait to hear Venus Roman." Celeste's eyes sparkle with excitement. "My shero."

"Ladies," Esmerelda says through the microphone on the stage, "please take your seats and let the GoddessFeast begin."

Welcome to The Biss Tribe

Suddenly the classical music stops and sexy Arabian dance music blasts. Then four Concierges push two giant genie bottles on wheels into the open space in the U-shaped table. A little door opens on each bottle, whose sides sparkle with a Moroccan-inspired pattern of gold and faux jewels. Men and women dressed as genies tumble out amidst poufs of orange and purple smoke.

The genies—whose skin is painted cobalt blue and emerald green and gold—look bewildered at first, then dramatically dance toward you and each woman, with exaggerated expressions and hand gestures of discovery and awe. They glitter in the soft sunshine in bejeweled bikini tops, harem pants with slits up the sides, gold turbans on the men and long ponytails on the women—all of whom have bare, chiseled abs and shapely shoulders.

"My Goddesses!" Biss exudes excitement from the stage. "Live your life as if your every wish is a command and the Universe is the genie who's here to grant your wishes. Especially around every form of Pleasure you can imagine."

Several women squeal with delight as the Concierges pour flat and sparkling water, wine and kombucha, and serve cocktails and mocktails according to each woman's preference.

The dancers pull brass genie lamps—the long kind with a handle at the back and a curvy spout at the front—from chains on their waistbelts. They dramatically dance close to the table, then hold a genie lamp in front of you and each woman, demonstrating how to rub the lamp without touching it. Then they hold each wishing lamp over the table, close enough for you to touch it.

"My Goddesses," Biss says, "imagine every day that you have the Power to rub the limitless genie lamp of the Universe and make your wishes come true. Do it now!"

You, like the other women, stroke your fingers along the sides of the genie lamps. Jewel-toned mist shoots from the tip.

Tuesday, Day 3

"Oh my Goddess!" Marla exclaims.

"That is so freaking cool!" Sammie adds as the women gasp and shriek.

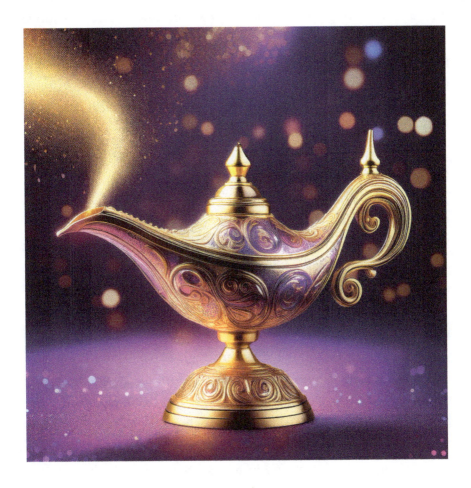

"Cool, man," Andi says, "but my life has been more like cutting myself on a tin can."

"Ladies," Biss says, "in the colorful mist of your imagination, know that anything is possible."

Each genie-dancer holds their palm in the colorful mist and pulls it out to reveal gold coins, jumbo jewels and mini cars, houses and trophies. They dramatically display the items for you.

"Everyone," Biss says, "say, 'I can do it, because I have the Power!'"

As you and the women say that in unison, the genies launch into a sexy group dance amidst colorful smoke and sensuous music. When it concludes, Biss says, "Now enjoy your meals and get ready for our very special speaker this evening, Venus Roman, co-founder of Husbands, Incorporated."

The Concierges serve each woman a platter holding a silver fondue pot with tiny forks and dipping items. They lift the lid on each woman's pot to reveal bubbling melted cheese or a non-dairy and/or vegan cheese for some.

"Let's give thanks," Biss says. "My Goddesses, let's close our eyes and give thanks to the infinite, divine powers for gifting us with this nourishment that fuels our minds, bodies and souls to activate our GoddessPleasure, so we can enjoy luscious lives that illuminate the world. And so it is spoken, and so it is done."

The women repeat a deep chorus of: "And so it is spoken, and so it is done."

Celeste spears a cube of sourdough bread and dips it into the pot, inhaling the aromatic steam, then pulling out the bread covered in stretchy orange cheese. "I am in heaven right now," she says before putting it in her mouth, closing her eyes and moaning.

Delaney dips small pieces of steam-softened broccoli into her fondue pot, and it's covered in melted Swiss, which she admires before savoring.

Kiki's platter holds cheese cubes that she dips and covers in more cheese.

"Isn't that overkill?" Andi asks, dipping a rye bread cube into her pot.

Kiki flashes a mischievous smile. "No, it's the definition of decadent. And I fucking love it." She sticks out her tongue in a sassy way at Andi, who chuckles.

Tuesday, Day 3

"A food-gasm once again," Zeusse says, dipping a garlic-buttered breadstick into her pot, biting its cheese-covered tip, and closing her eyes.

"Nobody talk to me right now," Sammie says playfully. "This is like literally better than sex."

"Well don't do this every day," Marla says, "or you'll blow up and never get your husband."

"Don't fat-shame me, bitch," Sammie quips, "while I make love to my cheese."

Kiki laughs.

"Damn." Zeusse stares at the food in awe as the string quartet plays sensuous music.

"Look at Venus Roman!" Celeste nods toward the other end of the U-shaped table where Venus is dining with Biss and Esmerelda. "She reminds me of Sharon Stone with the short blond hair."

"I love her strappy white dress," Sammie adds.

"And her diamond earrings," Marla says. "I can see them from here."

"That woman looks like she don't play," Celeste gushes. "I love how she graced her way through the hell-storm that her ex-husband and the protesters put her through when she went global with her company. Like, *Yawl can't touch this Goddess.*"

As several women laugh, Delaney smiles. "One of the tenured professors at my university actually married a man from Husbands, Incorporated. She wanted to be named department chair, and she thought that having the respectability and stability of a husband to take to our university functions would get her promoted."

"Did it?" Celeste asks.

"Yes, indeed it did," Delaney says. "She played the patriarchal game and got what she wanted. She also wanted someone who looked good and sounded intelligent—who could really deliver behind closed doors."

"Did he?" Bianca asks.

"Did he!" Delaney grins. "My poor friend didn't publish in any of the scholarly journals that year. She had no time to write, because they were always in bed. But she had the time of her life."

"I am swooning right now." Sunshine playfully holds the back of her wrist to her forehead.

"I think Venus is gonna light it up tonight," Zeusse says before enjoying another bite of a cheesy breadstick.

After awhile, the Concierges replace the fondue pots with small gold plates offering arugula greens in rich dressing shaped into a nest filled with a mound of seafood salad that glistens with luscious chunks of crab and lobster.

"Anyone with a shellfish allergy," Esmerelda announces, "will enjoy our culinary team's award-winning bean salad in your arugula nests."

"Man," Andi says, "I want to eat like this at home. Every day. But it's not realistic to live like this—"

"Whatever you say and believe," Celeste says, holding a chunk of crab with salad greens on her fork, "will be your reality. I'm done with reality. I'm with Kiki. I might get a tattoo of the word 'decadent' on my hand to remind me every damn day to be that and do that."

"Hell yeah!" Kiki smiles at Celeste, whose expression turns euphoric as she eats.

After the Concierges clear the salad plates, Bianca asks, "Did everyone see the private playroom with the toy box?"

"That chair with the mirror and light is whack," Marla says. "I'm way too embarrassed to look—"

"You have to!" Sammie spats. "It's our homework, and you of all people need to do that."

Tuesday, Day 3

Sunshine nods. "You should know what your body looks like, so if anything changes, you'll know to go to the doctor."

"A girl in my band masturbates in the mirror all the time," Jade says. "She says it turns her on and makes her feel more in touch with herself. She also has a mirror over her bed to watch when she's having sex a guy. She's such an exhibitionist and voyeur. I love her free spirit with zero hang-ups."

"What about them offering to help you learn the erotic devices?" Delaney asks.

"Ick factor," Sammie says. "I can figure that out myself."

"I can't," Andi says. "I don't know what the hell to do with all those plastic things. I need a crash course so I can make my future wife have a GoddessPleasure Awakening like none other."

"That's what's up," Zeusse says as the Concierges arrive with aromatic entrées that are covered by silver domes that have jeweled handles on top.

"Ladies," Esmerelda announces, "enjoy your entrées that are inspired by romantic cuisine from around the world. Each dish is carefully curated with ingredients that are aphrodisiacs. That means they stimulate emotional and physical desire and enhance Pleasure. Bon appetit!"

"Bring me the whole menu!" Marla says as her Concierge lifts the dome and says, "Angel hair pasta in garlic-tomato sauce with jumbo scallops pan-seared in truffle oil with a sprinkle of saffron." Marla looks ecstatic.

Delaney's Concierge lifts the dome over her plate and says, "Japanese-inspired Anago no Kabayaki, which is saltwater eel over ginger-fried rice with Tempura Shiitake."

Andi's Concierge reveals her meal and says, "Duck confit with a cherry balsamic reduction paired with fingerling potatoes and asparagus spears."

For Zeusse, her Concierge lifts the dome and says, "Basil and garlic-crusted baked oysters over pesto penne pasta drizzled with olive oil and garnished with artichokes."

Zeusse has a dreamy expression as she inhales the garlic and basil scents and ogles the artistic display of pasta surrounded by triangular artichoke leaves that are placed like green flower petals around the basil-specked pasta and golden-brown oysters.

As Concierge Jami lifts your dome and reveals your entrée, you savor the scents and enjoy the textures and tastes of each bite.

Goddess Feast Speaker: The Venus Roman Story

The Concierges serve desserts, which resemble mini erupting volcanos. Zeusse presses her spoon into a round chocolate Bundt Cake whose center holds a mound of vanilla ice cream dripping with hot fudge and sprinkled with pomegranate seeds.

Delaney eyes plump red strawberries stacked around a small bowl of melted dark chocolate for dipping. Kiki ogles a donut-shaped cherry pie with a scoop of pink ice cream in the center, drizzled with chocolate sauce and topped with whipped cream and a fresh cherry.

"This is so delicious," Celeste says, raising a spoonful of pecan pie and French vanilla ice cream toward her mouth, "I think I have an obscene expression on my face right now. But ask me if I care." She eats it, closes her eyes, and moans.

As you and the women enjoy your desserts, Biss heads to the stage.

"My Goddesses!" she says, wearing a shimmery purple bikini under a semi-sheer lace sleeveless dress that hugs her curves and sparkles with tiny rhinestones. Her hair is twisted up in a tumble

Tuesday, Day 3

of curls and held with a small sparkling purple tiara. "Are you loving this taste of the most luscious lifestyle you can imagine?"

The women cheer.

"Well, you ain't seen nothin' yet!" Biss says. "Just wait till you hear what our guest speaker did when she got sick and tired of being unsatisfied and oppressed!"

Biss gazes toward one end of the U-shaped table where she'd been dining with Esmerelda and Venus Roman. She glows as she looks at Venus, who remains seated.

"You're about to meet a woman who epitomizes GoddessPower and GoddessPleasure in every way," Biss says. "But first, let me tell you about Venus Roman. She wanted the American Dream, and she got it. It started when she was at the University of Michigan and met a young lawyer whose future was paved with gold. She married him in a big white wedding, soon got pregnant, and raised their twins in a beautiful suburban home with the proverbial white picket fence and life of luxury. She truly had it all, including a doting and devoted husband. So what could possibly go wrong?"

Biss looks playful. "Let's hear it from the Goddess herself, Venus Roman!"

As the women explode in applause, Venus stands and walks toward Biss's outstretched arms on the stage.

"We couldn't be more thrilled to have you here," Biss says as they embrace amidst ear-splitting cheers.

"It's my honor and privilege to join all of you," Venus says, making eye contact with you and all the women, who whisper about the fiery energy radiating from her eyes and aura.

"Please, Venus, take a seat." Biss motions toward a plush throne chair.

They sit with perfect posture, facing the women as you enjoy your desserts. The early sunset casts a pink hue over the terrace.

"So, Venus," Biss says, "take us to the night when you had your GoddessAwakening. When you knew that you were done with the marriage and wanted to do something bold to help women on a global scale."

Venus smiles. "First, I want to thank you, Biss, for inviting me here to talk with these Goddesses about Power and Pleasure."

"We're thrilled," Biss says as the women cheer.

"My GoddessAwakening," Venus says, making eye contact with you and each woman, "happened on a Valentine's Day when I was determined to rekindle the long-dead flames of romance and passion between me and my husband. Let me preface by saying that my libido was so blazing hot all the time, I would fantasize about the young men who landscaped our neighborhood, or worked out at my gym, or bagged my groceries at the market, or seemed to be everywhere, taunting my attention-starved mind and Pleasure-starved body. I felt like a live wire and desperately craved sex. But I would not commit adultery. I wanted my husband to want me as voraciously as he once had."

You and the women continue to savor your desserts as Venus talks.

"So, when our teenaged twins were away for the Valentine's Day weekend on a school trip, I got all dolled up in lingerie, filled the house with candles, had champagne waiting when he got home from work—"

Venus shakes her head. "But he hardly looked at me, and he smelled like some other bitch's perfume. We had to attend a gala later that night, where I played the role of smiling wife amongst many others doing the same, while our husbands engaged in the sport of woman-watching and even taking phone numbers from future playmates, right under our noses."

"I hate that feeling," Sunshine whispers.

Tuesday, Day 3

"Well, on this night, my husband's behavior was especially flagrant," Venus says, "and Raye saved me from losing it in front of everyone. Shortly thereafter, I divorced. Raye and I attended The Biss Tribe Retreat, where together we conceived our GoddessVision for Husbands, Incorporated. At the time, Raye had already curated a rotation of very desirable men who provided excellent and satisfying sex who also escorted her as a high-profile, powerful financial wizard to her many banquets, black tie galas and business trips."

Biss looks out at you and the women. "Raye Johnson was recently named one of the most influential and successful female financial advisors in America. You'll get the thrill of hearing her speak tomorrow at The GoddessTreasure Cave."

Venus adds, "Raye is one of the most bad ass women you'll ever meet. She brought the business brilliance to our company, and I brought the hunger and perspective of a woman whose American Dream had died. I was suffering from emotional neglect, dead love, and no sex, despite my best efforts to stay attractive, interesting and fun for my husband."

Bianca says with a disgusted tone, "Been there. Hated it." Several women echo her angst.

Biss acknowledges their pain with a nod, then turns back to Venus. "Venus, you transformed your pain into power, which inspired your business model. Can you describe it?"

"Husbands, Incorporated started with my belief, based on my personal experience, that monogamy is a myth," Venus says, "that humans are naturally curious sexual beings, that our sexuality is fluid and non-conforming to the conventions that we're taught from birth, and that men in particular are biologically hard-wired to spread their seed far and wide to continue the human race, while women are conditioned to mate for life to provide a stable environment for raising children while sadly clinging to the often-impossible fantasy of living happily ever after with her Prince Charming."

"Damn!" Zeusse exclaims. "She speaks the truth."

"Unfortunately," Sunshine says.

"Even those of us in good, stable marriages," Delaney says, nodding toward Celeste, "definitely go through our struggles where we want to call it quits."

"Amen to that," Celeste says. "But it makes us stronger in the end. I have no regrets on that. I have a good man."

A peaceful expression washes over Delaney's face as she says, "As do I."

Venus continues, "Our business model is also rooted in Raye's belief that true love is a lie, which speaks to her personal experience. Along with this are two beliefs that we share. First, you get excellent service for what you pay for. And second, the person in the marriage who holds the purse strings—typically the man—usually holds the Power, and with that Power, he dictates when or *if* the woman receives sexual Pleasure. Too often, after he's become bored with a traditional wife in bed, and he seeks the thrill of extramarital affairs, the devoted wife remains ignored and unsatisfied, as Raye and I were."

Venus radiates confidence as she says, "Our business model provides a luscious remedy for this all-too-common experience."

Biss turns to you and all the women. "This is all about turning your pain into Power! And being a bold innovator!" She draws her brows together and looks back at Venus. "Critics in the media have called you jaded, anti-family, anti-marriage and a deviant disruptor of societal norms."

Venus beams and sits up straighter. "I am all of that and more. I am also an eight-figure business owner with Raye, and we are ranked amongst the top 100 wealthiest women in the world.

Tuesday, Day 3

Thousands of men and women have benefited from their experiences in our company, and we're opening one new franchise per week in countries around the planet. So clearly the tremendous demand for our services, especially in the United States where half of traditional marriages end in divorce, speaks loudly and clearly for itself."

Marla and Sammie cheer and shout, "We love you, Venus!"

Venus beams. "Thank you, Goddesses."

She looks at Biss. "Now back to our business model. Our world headquarters are in a waterfront mansion in Detroit, where women from around the globe come to learn how to open a franchise and/or select their perfect mate. This selection process occurs during a visual extravaganza of men as they play in the pool, lounge on the yacht docked on the river, work out in the outdoor gym and mingle at receptions. Prior to that, we conduct extensive interviews with each woman to learn exactly what type of man and experience she's seeking."

"I love that," Biss says. "And you're not just talking about muscles with a certain hair, skin and eye color."

"Not at all," Venus says. "While each woman's ideal physical type is important, our marriages are much more than that."

"Marriages," Biss says, "that are not the norm."

"No, each marriage lasts only one year," Venus says. "The Husband signs a prenuptial agreement promising that if he performs his unique marital duties that each woman specifies in writing, he is entitled to a large financial pay-out when the marriage ends 12 months later in the U.S. territory of Guam, where the couple enjoys a sort of reverse honeymoon to establish the seven days of residency that are required to obtain a legal divorce there."

Biss smiles. "And the benefit of a legal, one-year marriage is what?"

Venus nods. "It's huge. Many women so profoundly dread the consequences of being labeled a slut or a whore or promiscuous or being accused of having loose morals and sleeping around, that they prefer what they perceive as the respectable status of having a husband. However, our clients do not want to commit for a lifetime, and they want guaranteed satisfaction in the bedroom, along with Power in the relationship."

Venus makes eye contact with each woman as she speaks. "When we pay for a service, we have control and influence over its quality and outcome. Like when you pay for a gourmet meal at an upscale restaurant, it comes with exquisite service and delicious food. The same applies for relationships. Except we can't buy people, and paying for sex is illegal in most states, while risky to your health and safety. Therefore, our business model provides what women want in a way that's legal, respectable and safe."

"Let's be clear," Biss says, "what is the typical demographic of your clients?"

"Most of them," Venus says, "are like myself and Raye. We fantasized about our wedding day as little girls, found our Prince Charming… put on the big white dress… played house, I had babies, Raye did not, but we both supported our husbands's careers…. then realized five, ten, fifteen or more years into it, that the white picket fence felt like prison bars… and our Prince Charming had turned into a frog!"

The women explode in laughter and boos.

"Then we realized," Venus says, "that we were locked in the castle tower with dishes and laundry, and me with diapers, playdates and homework, while Prince Charming was gallivanting off to conquer new damsels."

Groans of sadness and disappointment ripple around the table.

Tuesday, Day 3

"But this is not the case for all of our clients," Venus adds. "Many are in their early twenties. They've never been married and have no desire to do so in a traditional sense. These young female superstars are busy running businesses and traveling the world and doing things that our female ancestors—and our mothers for that matter—could never imagine doing. But these young women want companions, without the drama or the deceit or the risks posed by money-hungry lotharios."

Biss asks, "Do the marriages work out well for these women?"

"Yes," Venus says, "because they're used to having control, getting what they want, and protecting their assets. Marriages at Husbands, Inc. help ensure that."

Biss nods. "What are some things that can go wrong with these Husbands-for-hire?"

"That's what I want to know," Sunshine whispers.

"People are not robots," Venus says. "Whatever unresolved emotional issues a person brings to the marriage will come out, despite their best efforts to suppress them. For example, we had one client whose excruciating insecurity was triggered by her belief that her worth to a man was strictly measured by her appearance. She had no self-worth- and no idea who she was on the inside."

"Poor girl." Kiki shakes her head and eats the cherry from her dessert.

"I can relate," Jade adds.

"So all this unraveled in the marriage," Venus continues. "Thankfully, her Husband recognized this, and went above and beyond the call of duty to apply his skills as an experienced lady's man and kind-hearted person. He helped her see her worth on the inside."

"Did they live happily ever after?" Sammie asks.

Welcome to The Biss Tribe

"That's not the mission of Husbands, Incorporated," Venus says with a sharp tone. "Our client left the year-long marriage as a woman who found her Power within, much like you do here in The Biss Tribe. She took with her the unexpected gift of transformation. Our Husband benefitted too, because the experience unveiled a skillset that he didn't know he had."

Phyllis raises her hand. "Do you cater to women who have children?"

Venus shakes her head. "No. Raye and I decided from the start that we did not want to introduce the Husbands into situations where a single mother is bringing a man—even though he is thoroughly vetted by us with a criminal background check and extensive mental and physical health evaluations—into a home with children. It's too complicated and risky for a long list of reasons."

Phyllis looks and sounds aggravated: "Reasons like what? It seems like you're discriminating against moms who just want love."

Venus shakes her head and speaks with a firm tone while looking at Phyllis. "Our Husbands are trained to be perfect companions for adventurous living, sex partners for unprecedented satisfaction, and escorts for women who attend high profile parties, corporate events and formal affairs. Our Husbands are not trained to interact with children or to navigate the many dynamics of children that include jealous or hostile biological fathers, custody issues, domestic duties, childcare, school responsibilities, etcetera."

Phyllis crosses her arms. "I don't think that's fair. Single moms need love, too."

"They absolutely do," Venus says. "We encourage them to find love the traditional way. Our model would cause emotional trauma for children who become attached to a Husband who leaves after

Tuesday, Day 3

one year. Again, our business model unapologetically caters to women who do not have small children or teenagers in the home, and who are free to enjoy an adult-only relationship."

Tension hangs in the air as Phyllis sulks.

Biss diffuses it with an upbeat tone as she asks, "Venus, tell us about the financial aspect of a fantasy marriage with Husbands, Inc."

"We cater to affluent women who have the resources to pay the financial settlement at the end of the marriage," Venus says. "Fortunately, many of our wealthy clients contribute to The Husbands, Inc. Foundation, which provides scholarships for women who typically could not afford our experience, so that they can enjoy the Husband of their choice for one year. The costs are high, because they include the significant fees for our services to conduct the extensive interview process and provide the customized training for each client's selected Husband."

"Training!" Biss exclaims. "Tell us about *that!*"

Venus beams, glancing out at you and all the women. "Ladies! How many of you have a fantasy man? Say, a rock star? A football player? A banker? Or a fashion model?"

The women cheer.

"At Husbands, Inc.," Venus says, "we have an acting academy where Husbands are trained to the unique specifications that each woman requests. The men also learn etiquette and lovemaking techniques that guarantee satisfaction."

Several women cheer as Sunshine says, "That sounds heavenly."

Biss smiles and says playfully, "Speaking of specifications, the Husbands have to fulfill certain physical requirements."

Venus nods. "Oh, yes. They need stamina for at least 30 minutes of continuous and vigorous intercourse, without medicine, and they need to come to us with a penis that measures a minimum length and girth, unless a woman requests otherwise."

Biss nods, "What about same-sex couples?"

"We recently expanded to offer LGBTQ+ marriages that follow the same model," Venus says.

"That's what's up," Zeusse says.

The evening sunshine casts an ever-softening golden glow over Biss, Venus and everyone on the terrace.

"Alright, Venus, let's get to the juicy stuff," Biss says. "You had a ravenous appetite for men when you left your marriage. Did Husbands, Inc. satisfy it?"

Venus glows so brightly, it's like a star exploded inside her. "I hardly have words to describe the Pleasure that I experience every day. I remember the first time I took a lover—I don't have to marry them because I own the company—but I have had several Husbands and will tell you my current status in a little while. The first time gifted me with my GoddessPleasure Awakening. I learned that term here in The Biss Tribe. Well, ladies, with this extremely energetic and talented young man, I felt sensations in my body that I didn't know were possible. I had thought that the sex early on with John was great. But I met him during college and had never been with another man."

Venus grips the sides of her chair and leans back as if a strong wind is blowing toward her. "Ladies! It blew my mind. And my first thought was, *I want women everywhere to experience extreme Pleasure like this!* So I set off on my mission to do exactly that. We now have 44 franchises around the world. Josephine DuJardin opened the first one in Paris, and I'm going there next week to celebrate its expansion to an office in Nice in the South of France."

"Congratulations!" Biss says. "What's your advice to our Goddesses here tonight?"

"No more suffering!" Venus declares. "You deserve love!"

The women cheer.

Tuesday, Day 3

"You deserve to feel desired!" Venus proclaims. "You deserve the gift of being with someone who treats you like a Goddess, for 365 days a year!"

"Yes!" several women cheer and clap.

Then Biss asks, "Venus, can we do a Q&A?"

"Of course."

Sunshine raises her hand. "What if the woman and the man fall in love for real, and want the marriage to continue when the year is up?"

Venus smiles. "This is one of the most common questions I hear from people who are curious about Husbands, Inc. It *does* happen that our couples sometimes fall in love for real. When this happens, the spouses sign a legal agreement that nullifies the clauses stating that the marriage will end after 12 months. Also nullified is the obligation to provide the payment that was promised in the prenup. Then the couple is free to live happily ever after. Should they divorce at a later date, they would proceed without any of the protections or involvement of our company."

Sunshine asks, "Do you keep analytics on how many of those real marriages last or end in divorce?"

"No, but based on anecdotal evidence, and thanks to our extraordinary matchmaking process, the marriages remain solid and strong."

Celeste raises her hand. "Venus, did you marry Rex? I remember he came along and tried to convince you that true love and monogamy can be real when you find your soul mate."

Venus beams. "Rex is truly my soul mate. I did go through with a marriage to him. Whether it's a Husbands, Inc.-style marriage or a conventional one 'til death do us part, that's classified." Venus winks at Celeste.

"Either way, you're my shero," Celeste says, standing and applauding, which inspires the other women to do the same.

"I can't thank you enough," Venus tells Celeste, "for sharing that."

Suddenly sexy music booms; 11 cowboys and 11 cowgirls strut into the open area between the table and the stage. They move in perfect synchronicity, and their skin—which ranges from creamy white to coffee bean black—glistens as if oiled.

DJ Panther in the elevated booth blasts a medley of sexy songs like "Pony" by Ginuwine and "Lady Marmalade" by Christina Aguilera with P!nk, Mya and Lil' Kim, along with sultry hits by Megan Thee Stallion, Cardi B, Madonna and Donna Summer.

The shirtless, muscular men are wearing rhinestone-studded cowboy hats, cowboy boots and faded jeans and silver leather chaps with fringe down the sides, while the women are similarly dressed with bejeweled denim bikini tops whose silver fringe sways over their bare abs and backs.

They do a provocative line dance, then pair off with erotic moves that rouse loud cheers and gasps from the women as Biss and Venus watch with delight from the stage.

"That is pure fire!" Kiki says as some women's jaws drop and others clap to the beat. "I want performances like that at my club."

The genie dancers twirl out from behind the stage to join the cowboys and cowgirls in an erotic dancing extravaganza.

Sunshine eyes one of the genie dancers. "That one is exactly my type." She looks up at the darkening pink sky as a fiery orange disk of the setting sun glows through pine trees at one edge of the terrace. "I declare and command," she says to the sky, "that my husband will show up looking like him or better, and shower me with love and Pleasure like I've never known."

Tuesday, Day 3

Several women witness Sunshine's declaration to the universe. Jade leans toward her and says, "And so it is spoken, and so it is done." Then they do the GoddessGreeting and turn back to watch the dancers. Sunshine delights in watching the genie-costumed man who has buff muscles, bronze skin and long, dark hair that sways over his back as he dances. She catches his eye, he winks, and she smiles.

Biss and Venus stand and step down into the frenzy of dancers. "My Goddesses!" Venus shouts. "Everybody get up and dance!"

You and the women spring up and join the dancers as the sultry music beats louder and faster. Sunshine shimmies close to her genie dream man, beaming with delight as he takes her hands over her head and spins her around, gazing down at her with passion burning in his eyes.

Jade dances with a cowboy and a cowgirl, while Zeusse and a voluptuous female genie get their groove on. Kiki jumps on the back of a cowboy, playfully kicks his sides like he's a horse, and swirls his hat around in the air. Multiple cowboys dance with Bianca, who's gleefully swaying her arms, lost in the music and the joyous energy engulfing the mass of people on the terrace.

Marla and Sammie dance and shriek as the cowboys, cowgirls and genies slink and slide with perfect precision through the group, stopping to dance with each woman, who lights up under their delighted gazes.

The sun sets, the sky goes dark, the mini-Moroccan lanterns strung around the terrace glow with orange, pink, yellow, purple and blue light, DJ Panther blasts sexy songs and euphoric expressions sweep across the women's faces.

Biss makes her way through the group, beaming at you and declaring, "Celebrate your GoddessPleasure every day!"

Welcome to The Biss Tribe

Discussing Aphrodisiacs in the Hot Springs

Sweating and feeling euphoric from dancing, you and the women make your way to the hot springs.

The almost-full silver moon glows huge against the black sky amidst sparkling stars, casting a lavender glow over the steaming water. The large oval pool is surrounded by a smooth rock patio and several raised fire pits whose orange-yellow flames create a soft haze around the women and the steam.

"My Goddesses," Biss says with Venus at her side as they stand by the water, "it's time to enjoy a full-body massage—" she motions toward several women, including Bianca, who are getting rubbed with oil on massage tables by masseuses amidst the fire pits "—or take a soothing soak in our steaming mineral bath."

"How do we know the water won't burn us?" Sammie asks. "I mean, is it boiling hot?"

Biss dips her toes into the dark water. "The hot springs here at The GoddessPleasure Tent on Infinity Mountain remain a consistent 101 degrees Fahrenheit and are electronically monitored around the clock. The water naturally bubbles up from the earth into this pool that we built to enhance your soaking experience. If the temperature exceeds 104 degrees, our high-tech, underground sensors will instantly alert us and we'll immediately get out of the water. You are Class number 88 in The Biss Tribe, and every woman before you has had a safe, rejuvenating experience here in the mineral baths."

A woman in a flowing white gown takes a seat at a harp near the pool. Her strums create enchanting music.

"That is so beautiful." Marla closes her eyes and sways. "So soothing."

Biss and Venus remove their dresses, which Concierges carry away, and they step down the stone steps into the pool.

Tuesday, Day 3

"My Goddesses," Biss says, "come in. Sit on the big, smooth rocks around the edges. They form an underwater bench." Biss and Venus sit as the chest-high water bubbles around them.

"Oh my God, this feels so good," Sunshine exclaims, sitting beside Esmerelda. "It's tingly."

You and the other women place your clothing on nearby benches and get in. Once you're settled onto the comfortable underwater rock bench, the Concierges arrive, serving each woman's favorite cocktail, mocktail, wine, water or other beverage.

"This is the life, man," Andi says, sipping a gin and tonic.

"I love that smell," Celeste says, inhaling deeply. "Like wet rocks and earth and something else—"

"Ladies," says Esmerelda, who's sitting beside Biss, "you're soaking in mineral water that naturally contains a high concentration of lithium, which has a calming effect on your body and boosts your mood. It's also infused with the mystical healing powers of the crystal beds under Infinity Mountain. So you'll sleep like a baby tonight."

"With a smile on our faces," Kiki says, "after we play with our toys."

"Yes!" Biss says.

"Venus," Celeste asks, "will you tell us more about your daily life?"

"Cheers to that!" Kiki raises her martini, inspiring the women to clink your glasses together and sip. "You are the O.G. Original Goddess. Or Original Gangster! For what you do for women."

"Truth!" Zeusse says with a smile.

Venus's blue eyes sparkle as she says, "I'll take that. Thank you. My greatest two thrills every day are the physical Pleasure that I experience exactly as I desire, and the excitement that I see in women's eyes when they tell me that they've had their GoddessPleasure Awakenings with their Husbands."

Venus beams, then says, "I actually don't have words to describe the thrill of providing our service that gives this life-changing gift to women who have felt tossed out, overlooked, neglected, unsatisfied and downright depressed. A lot of these women experience real Pleasure for the first time in their lives, and some are in their forties, fifties and even sixties."

Venus looks at Biss as the water gurgles around them. "Biss, you and I actually provide a similar service, because we both help women awaken to the infinite possibilities of life when we disrupt the status quo and create a better way."

Zeusse raises her glass. "Toast to disrupting the status quo!"

You and the women clink your glasses.

Delaney asks, "Venus, how did you stay sane during the protests and legal harassment that your ex-husband was orchestrating to try and stop you?"

"That's a great question," Venus says. "Because if your GoddessMission is something that disrupts the status quo, like Husbands, Incorporated is, you *will* face opposition. Threats. Protests. Legal challenges. It can feel like a nightmare."

"Cripe," Andi says.

"So to answer your question," Venus says, looking at Delaney, "I stayed sane by keeping my GoddessVision foremost in my mind, 24/7. No matter what was happening in my physical reality, my Supernatural Self was dwelling on my vision of resolving all the legal problems and proceeding with our global expansion as Raye and I had planned."

"I love this!" Biss says as the harp player hits dramatic notes.

"And it worked," Venus says. "My GoddessVision triumphed over the evil plots that John, the protesters and everybody else used to try and stop us. So, beautiful Goddesses, believe and never stop believing, no matter what's happening. You were blessed with your GoddessVision for a reason. That's your calling. Your assignment. Do everything possible to make it happen!"

Tuesday, Day 3

"We are all in!" Marla exclaims, raising her champagne flute as Sammie does the same beside her.

After you and the women toast, Sammie says with a dreamy tone, "That harp music, the champagne, this hot water... I feel like I'm floating in heaven right now."

"You and me both," Kiki says, looking around as the dancing flames reflect on the black water and illuminate the steam. "This is inspiring me to add a water element to my club. It's so sexy and relaxing."

"Look at you, Kiki!" Marla says. "You came here with no idea what to do with your life, and you got your GoddessVision."

"Crystal clear," Kiki says. She turns to Biss. "Biss! I want to say thank you, but those two words are way too small to tell you how I really feel." She looks up at the moon. "Like, over the moon with excitement."

Biss beams at Kiki and says, "You can do it, Goddess, because *you* have the power!"

The women are silent for a moment as the harp music plays.

"Venus," Zeusse asks, "can you tell us what you do for self-care when you're stressed out?"

"Orgasms." Venus flashes a mellow smile.

Zeusse nods. "That's what's up."

Venus adds, "Pleasure sweeps me away from angst, into an oasis of bliss. When I'm with my lover who knows exactly how to please me, I envision the Pleasure washing away whatever had been troubling me. I also use Orgasmic Visualization to channel and focus my sex energy, the energy of creation, into the best outcome to resolve the problem."

"So that really works?" Andi asks.

"Like magic," Venus says.

"And for those of you who need scientific proof," Venus says, "studies show that orgasms cause chemical reactions in our bodies that boost our mental and physical health. Orgasms flood our bodies with the Pleasure hormone oxytocin, which neutralizes the stress hormone cortisol. And we all know cortisol is a killer."

Venus looks at you and each woman. "Ladies, do you hear me? We can create in our bodies a chemical that kills cortisol to save ourselves from the sickness and even strokes that high levels of stress can cause. That's motivation enough to have as many orgasms as possible, along with the immense Pleasure that they bring."

Marla lets out a nervous giggle. "Hashtag 'I hope so.' This is all aspirational for me right now."

The Concierges appear, kneeling at the sides of the pool to offer silver bowls of nuts, strawberries, olives, foie gras on crackers, tiny cups of pomegranate seeds and chocolates.

"Speaking of chemical reactions in the body," Esmerelda says, "enjoy these snacks that are all proven aphrodisiacs."

Andi asks, "Are aphrodisiacs just a placebo effect? Is it that we think these foods enhance romance, so they do? Or is it really scientific?"

"It's both," Esmerelda says. "Aphrodisiac foods are either shaped like sex organs, have sensuous tastes and textures, or contain vitamins and other nutrients that arouse our minds and bodies."

"I definitely feel a difference when I eat oysters," Zeusse says.

"Chocolate for me," Sunshine adds. "Whether it's scientific or not, I know how I feel. And that's what matters."

Biss raises her champagne flute. "Cheers to what Sunshine just said. My Goddesses, Pleasure is all about what *you* like, and how you like it!"

You and the women toast in a loud clink of glasses and laughter.

"OK chicklets," Kiki says, climbing out of the pool and dripping water on the stone patio. "It's time to go play in my toybox!"

Tuesday, Day 3

As her Concierge puts a hooded robe made of thick towel fabric on her and ties the belt, she looks at him. "And I want *you* to be my playmate."

"At your service, madame," her Concierge says.

Kiki smiles at Biss and Venus, then at you and all the women. "If you hear obscene sounds coming from my tent, you'll know I'm having a really good time!"

Marla laughs. "Hashtag aspirational for me."

"Have the *best* time!" Biss says as Kiki and her Concierge walk away.

Marla says, "I want my Concierge to help me, too."

"I'm so proud of you, bitch!" Sammie says. "I want to hear all about it in the morning. I'll be solo as a preview of the coming year."

Andi nods. "I need my Concierge to show me how to do stuff, so my wife won't think I'm a fumbling loser. Hey Biss, thanks for pairing me up with a femme type who gets me."

"We aim to please here in The Biss Tribe," Biss says.

"Biss," Zeusse says, "can we hook up with the dancers?"

Jade high-fives Zeusse and says, "I was wondering the same thing!"

"Yes," Biss says. "You may. However, it's extremely important that you do the *PowerJournal* exercises tonight in relation to your self-exploration with the light and mirror, and experiments with the different types of stimulation with the devices in your toyboxes."

"Understood," Zeusse says, quickly stepping out of the water along with Jade. Their Concierges place robes on them before they hurry toward the dance floor.

"My Goddesses," Biss says, "hold nothing back tonight. It's all about *you!* You can do it, because *you* have the Power to enjoy Pleasure!"

Welcome to The Biss Tribe

Time for Self-Exploration

You return to your private tent, with or without your Concierge or a dancer, and venture into the playroom where the lounge chair, light and mirror await. You proceed to explore, as guided by your own curiosity and desire. Then you write about it in your *PowerJournal*.

If this is your first time using a mirror to see yourself between your legs, what are you first impressions?

_____

_____

_____

_____

Describe your emotions as you looked at yourself from this angle. Fear? Shame? Curiosity? Regret that it's taken this long?

_____

_____

_____

_____

Tuesday, Day 3

If this is not your first time using a mirror to see yourself between your legs, what are your impressions about any changes you may see due to age, hair growth or removal, or ideas about how you "should" appear down there?

_____

_____

_____

_____

_____

Toy Time

Next, it's time to explore the toy chest that's stocked with stimulating devices. Experiment with them to discover which ones you like most and write about your experiences. Indicate whether you prefer those that vibrate or not, as well as size and intensity.

Suction devices _____

The Rabbit _____

The Doxy Wand _____

Butt plugs _____

Dildos _____

Others _____

Welcome to The Biss Tribe

Dear Goddess Reader:

You can replicate this private self-exploration and experimentation with toys to discover what you enjoy most. Write about your experiences here and fill in the lines above. If you feel resistant to this, describe why.

_____

_____

_____

_____

_____

You have the Power to decide how you'll incorporate Pleasure into your life, so write three ways you can easily do that every day.

_____

_____

_____

_____

_____

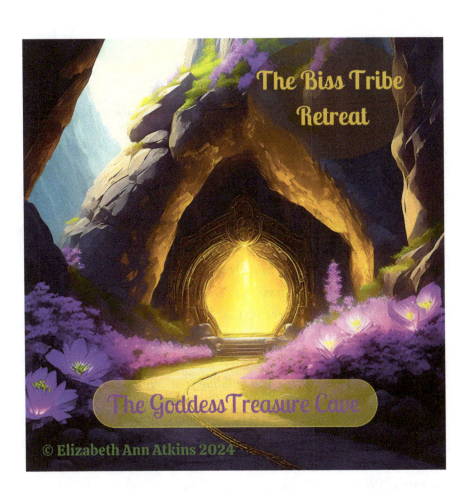

Welcome to The Biss Tribe

Continue Your Transformation on Infinity Mountain

Dear Goddess Reader:

Tomorrow, you'll travel up Infinity Mountain to the next Activation Station. Here's the schedule:

Sunday: The Biss Tribe Inn
Monday: The GoddessPower Pyramid
Tuesday: The GoddessPleasure Tent
Wednesday: The GoddessTreasure Cave
Thursday: The GoddessWarrior Fortress
Friday: The GoddessPeace Garden
Saturday: The GoddessPower Studios to record your personal podcast, followed by the Coronation at SeaGoddess Castle, then the GoddessFeast and evening cruise on Sea-Goddess yacht.
Sunday: Fly home to begin building your empire.

Two months from now, you'll return to The Biss Tribe to begin bi-monthly GoddessLife Intensives that give you guidance and advanced trainings on each of the five foundations of Power, Pleasure, Prosperity, Protection and Peace.

These four-day Intensives conclude with a training and celebration to mark the one-year anniversary of your entrée into The Biss Tribe and your GoddessLife.

You can do this, Goddess, because *you* have the power!

Tuesday, Day 3

Stay Connected and Inspired in the Goddess RoundTable Community

Don't stop your transformation and inspiration when you finish this book and wait for the next one.

You can get your daily dose of GoddessPower when you join my online community, The Goddess RoundTable. As a member, you'll:

- Enjoy a weekly energy cleanse, guided meditation and lively conversation about how to find your Peace and Power.

- Learn rituals and manifestation techniques that can make magic happen in your life.

- Continue your ascent into your GoddessLife amongst a safe, supportive sisterhood of diverse women from across America and beyond.

- Get discounts on private, one-on-one GoddessPower Coaching where I help you create and sustain a daily self-care regimen that includes healthier eating, exercise that you love, a spiritual practice (if desired), mindset shifts and lifestyle improvements that help you put yourself first, and the accountability that you need to make your GoddessLife your new reality. I want to help you level up so dramatically that every day you declare, "I've never felt better!"

- Get discounts for my Women Writing Books program to compose your novel, memoir or business book in my virtual book coaching program that births best-selling authors.

- Get discounts on my virtual and in-person retreats. Goddess RoundTable members get priority and exclusive entrée into my events and programs.

- Get automatically entered in my free give-away of a private, 45-minute coaching session ($300 value) to Activate Your GoddessPower. During this virtual experience, we'll: explore where you feel powerless; describe your GoddessVision and GoddessLife; do an energy cleanse and guided meditation to get guidance from Spirit on the action steps you need to take to step through your GoddessGateway; and discuss a daily action plan for you to use the four GoddessPower Activation Tools to manifest your dream life.

When you join The GoddessPower RoundTable, you commit to making the rest of your life, the best of your life. You can do it, Goddess, because *you* have the power!

Join us at TheGoddessPowerShow.com.

The Biss Tribe: Where You Celebrate Your GoddessCoronation

Each book has an accompanying *PowerJournal*.

1. PowerJournal to Activate Your GoddessPower
2. PowerJournal to Activate Your GoddessPleasure
3. PowerJournal to Activate Your GoddessProsperity
4. PowerJournal to Activate Your GoddessProtection
5. PowerJournal to Activate Your GoddessPeace

Books in The Biss Tribe Series

Available at TwoSistersWriting.com.

1. The Biss Tribe: Where You Activate Your GoddessPower
2. The Biss Tribe: Where You Activate Your GoddessPleasure
3. The Biss Tribe: Where You Activate Your GoddessProsperity
4. The Biss Tribe: Where You Activate Your GoddessProtection
5. The Biss Tribe: Where You Activate Your GoddessPeace
6. The Biss Tribe: Where You Activate Your GoddessCoronation

Roster

The Biss Tribe Class #88

Marla Santos—25, a social media influencer and co-founder of a skincare line with her best friend, Sammie Smithville.

Appearance: almond-shaped eyes, brown sugar-hued skin and a mane of straight black hair.

Background: grew up in Los Angeles in a large, Filipino-American family led by her father, a pastor.

Lives: in Miami, Florida, with Sammie.

Why she's here: To liberate herself from her parents's brainwashing that has guilted and shamed her to fear sex to the point that she's never had sex or an orgasm.

Goal: Expand her businesses to launch her skincare line, and get on the Forbes 30 Under 30 List, earning high seven figures.

Sammie Smithville—25, social media influencer and co-founder of a skincare line with her best friend, Marla Santos.

Appearance: Long, pin-straight blonde hair, blue eyes, vanilla skin and glossy pink Betty Boop lips.

Background: Grew up in Savannah, Georgia, in a wealthy family.

Lives: In Miami, Florida, with Marla.

Why she's here: To free herself from a destructive cycle of dating disappointments and man addiction that make her anxious and unhappy.

Goal: Expand her businesses to launch her skincare line, and get on the Forbes 30 Under 30 List, earning high seven figures.

Kiki Khalil—24, a friend of Marla and Sammie.

Appearance: Glassy, almond-hued skin, plump lips, thick black lashes, platinum-tipped brunette hair, and a slim, petite build.

Background: Grew up in an Arab American family in Dearborn, Michigan.

Lives: In Miami, Florida, with her brother and his wife.

Why she's here: To find herself.

Goal: Figure out her life purpose.

Zeusse—30, retired WNBA champion.

Appearance: 6'4" tall with an athletic build; cosmetic-free skin that's as rich and smooth as coffee beans; long, skinny dreadlocks; and wide-set eyes that convey wisdom and an "old soul" energy.

Background: Grew up with her father in Harlem, New York, and summered on her grandparents's farm in Alabama.

Lives: In a brownstone in Harlem.

Why she's here: To find the same courage and confidence that she has on the basketball court, in the business world.

Tuesday, Day 3

Goal: To strategize how to open and sustain a global franchise of girls basketball academies.

Jade Rogers—35, office worker and guitarist in a girl band, The Star Chix.

Appearance: Tattoos of green vines sprouting blue flowers and Greek goddess busts adorn her thin, milky-white arms. Blue eyeliner accentuates her hazel eyes and round, slightly plump face. She has pink hair.

Background: Grew up in an affluent White family in suburban Chicago, Illinois.

Lives: In a loft downtown Chicago.

Why she's here: To free herself from her parents's belief that she can't make a career of being a music artist.

Goal: To leave her corporate job and travel the world with her girl band.

Sunshine Bylilly—44, a struggling life coach and self-described narcissist magnet.

Appearance: Wears her dark hair in a high ponytail that showcases her caramel complexion and large, dark eyes highlighted by perfect black-winged liner and thick, natural lashes. She wears a sterling silver hummingbird pendant on her turquoise-beaded, choker-style necklace.

Background: Raised by her grandmother in the Navajo Nation in Santa Fe, New Mexico.

Lives: In a house she inherited from her grandmother in Santa Fe.

Why she's here: To find her self-worth and belief in herself.

Goal: To create a life coaching center called The Turquoise Experience that hires Indigenous women entrepreneurs while earning a seven-figure income. Also wants to find a loving, devoted husband.

Bianca Hernandez—47, a therapist at a mental health clinic specializing in girls and young women with anxiety. Uses a wheelchair after a car accident and has ADHD.

Appearance: Her turquoise hair matches her braces and the birds and flowers in her large tattoo of Mexican painter Frida Kahlo. With clear, peaches-and-cream skin and a silver scar on her cheek, she sparkles with rhinestones that she applies to her clothing, in her crystal bracelets and in a tiny Mexican flag pendant necklace.

Background: Raised in San Diego, California, by parents who own a restaurant.

Lives: In a condo in San Diego.

Why she's here: To find peace of mind and to focus on finishing what she starts.

Goal: To open a nonprofit called Amy's Oasis, a girls's enrichment center, to honor a patient who chose suicide after she didn't get into Harvard like her parents wanted.

Celeste Williams—54, CEO of a prominent company who's burned out by a demanding career while being a wife, mother of two sons, active in her faith community and caretaker of two parents with dementia.

Tuesday, Day 3

Appearance: Close-cropped, peroxide-blonde waves and a bronze complexion that glows like sunshine beaming through a jar of molasses. Her light brown eyes sparkle despite puffy under-eye bags obscured by concealer. Her blingy clothes and diamond wedding ring reflect her affluence.

Background: Raised in Detroit, Michigan.

Lives: In a beautiful home in an affluent Detroit suburb.

Why she's here: To learn how to make self-care a top priority after stress caused an agonizing eczema outbreak.

Goal: To leave her corporate CEO position and open a bakery and café, Celeste's Sweet Shop.

Andi Sullivan—61, coming out as gay on a mission to follow her dreams after a life dictated by her family.

Appearance: Thick with a masculine build and clothing style, she has an oval, cosmetic-free face distinguished by thick brows, gray eyes and freckled beige skin with tiny lines extending from the outer corners of her eyes when she smiles. Her chestnut-brown hair is shaved bald on one side and falls in a straight chop toward her chin on the other. She wears multiple silver hoop earrings and rings.

Background: Grew up Worchester, Massachusetts, in a large Irish American family that founded a successful chain of hardware stores. She lived her parents's expectations to marry a man, have kids, and work in the family business.

Lives: In her own house in her hometown.

Welcome to The Biss Tribe

Why she's here: To leave the family business and to find the courage to live on her own terms.

Goal: To open her beachfront art studio and to find a wife.

Delaney Cohen—74, an Ivy League university professor who is in a long-term marriage.

Appearance: She resembles the actress Meryl Streep but with curly, silver shoulder-length hair parted on one side and tucked behind an ear. She wears simple silver jewelry and dresses with an artsy, flowy-linen vibe.

Background: Grew up on New York's Upper East Side, in a Jewish family with a disapproving mother.

Lives: On a country estate near Princeton, New Jersey, with her husband.

Why she's here: To find inner peace and self-love so that she feels that despite her many accomplishments, she is enough just as she is.

Goal: To explore new possibilities for the next 25 years as she strives to live to a healthy 100 years old and beyond.

Tuesday, Day 3

The Biss Tribe Team

Biss—Founder of The Biss Tribe, where she leads life-changing retreats and teaches all the tools that have enabled her to transform from the inside out and create her dream life. A best-selling author, publisher, podcaster and multimedia journalist.

Appearance: Curly yellow hair, suntanned French vanilla skin, green eyes, athletic curves. She wears colorful clothing, crystal jewelry and lots of sparkle.

Background: Grew up in Michigan in a loving, multiracial family.

Lives: In The Biss Tribe Inn, at SeaGoddess Castle and in other residences.

Why she's here: To follow her GoddessMission.

Goal: To continue her divine life assignment to activate the infinite power in women everywhere and thus make the world a better place.

Esmerelda—Age unknown. Retreat leader, yogi, singer and sound bowl artist.

Appearance: With trim, toned muscles, her skin is so dewy and smooth, it reminds you of melted milk chocolate. Her blue eyes glow brightly from the luminescent contours of her face. Snow-white swirls of hair cascade down her back. It's impossible to tell her age or her ethnicity, and she radiates mesmerizing authority and warmth.

Background: Grew up in New Orleans, Louisiana.

Lives: In The Biss Tribe Inn and at SeaGoddess Castle.

Why she's here: She transformed in The Biss Tribe and never left.

Goal: Helping women experience healing and success.

Panther—Executive Assistant and DJ. Tall with jet-black-hair and a sparkling nose ring.

Vee—The bus driver and an assistant. Her emerald-green hair matches the colorful mermaids tattooed on her arms.

Concierges—The personal assistants each assigned to a Biss Tribe retreat-goer.

About the Author

Elizabeth Ann Atkins

Elizabeth's renegade spirit to blaze her own trails in life and love springs from her parents's scandalous union after her father—a Roman Catholic Priest who was French, English and Native American—left the church to marry a Black woman 25 years younger during the turbulent 1960s.

Their defiance of racial and religious conventions—all in the name of love—inspired Elizabeth as a multiracial woman to write herself into American literature with novels *White Chocolate, Dark Secret,* and *Twilight* with Billy Dee Williams, all published by the Tor/Forge imprint at St. Martin's Press.

Then, after a fairytale wedding and a nightmare divorce, Elizabeth's disillusionment with dating and traditional relationships inspired her to write an erotic trilogy, *Husbands, Incorporated*, about a company that provides legal, fantasy marriages that give women immense power and pleasure. The series is written under Elizabeth's pen name of Sasha Maxwell. Sasha's next book is *Eleven Men.*

To amplify messages of peace and empowerment, Elizabeth and her sister, author Catherine M. Greenspan, co-founded Two Sisters Writing & Publishing® in 2016, first publishing their own

Welcome to The Biss Tribe

fiction and non-fiction books that celebrate colorblind love and self-identity.

They have since published more than 50 books, mostly against-the-odds success stories by diverse authors from across America. Their authors include former Detroit Mayor Dennis Archer, the former president of the American Red Cross, judges, lawyers, physicians, surgeons, healers, executives and motivational speakers.

Two Sisters published their mother's book, *The Triumph of Rosemary: a Memoir* by Judge Marylin E. Atkins, which was developed into a screenplay with the goal of creating a Hollywood feature film.

Most recently, Elizabeth co-authored *Healing Religious Hurts: Stories & Tips to Find Love and Peace* and *Joyously Free: Stories & Tips to Live Your Truth as LGBTQ+ People, Parents and Allies* by Elizabeth Ann Atkins and Joanie Lindenmeyer.

Learn more and order books at TwoSistersWriting.com.

The Biss Tribe: Where You Activate Your GoddessPower by Elizabeth Ann Atkins is the first in a series of books that aim to awaken and empower women everywhere.

The books echo themes that Elizabeth writes and speaks about at TheGoddessPowerShow.com, which links to her podcast, *The Goddess Power Show with Elizabeth Ann Atkins®*. The show's mission is to explore sometimes taboo topics to inspire people to live bigger, better and bolder and manifest their hearts's wildest desires.

You can watch episodes on the YouTube channel for *The GoddessPower Show*. And you can listen to episodes on Apple Podcasts, Spotify, iHeart radio, and wherever you listen to podcasts. TheGoddessPowerShow.com provides links to all of the above, as well as the blog.

Elizabeth also co-hosts an Emmy-nominated TV show about mental health. *MI Healthy Mind* airs every Sunday on networks across Michigan and two episodes that Elizabeth hosted—interviewing a human trafficking survivor and people who became "wounded healers" by using their pain to help others—were nominated for Emmy Awards. Please visit MIHealthyMind.com and watch nine years's worth of episodes on YouTube.

Elizabeth's education laid the foundation for her career as a best-selling author, award-winning print journalist, Emmy-nominated TV show host, speaker, podcaster and publisher.

She earned a Bachelor of Arts degree as an English Literature major at the University of Michigan, where she began her journalism career as a reporter and editor at the campus newspaper, *The Michigan Daily*.

Then she earned a Master of Science degree from the Columbia University Graduate School of Journalism in New York City, where she focused on broadcast news and international reporting. During that time, she had a part-time job as a copy clerk at *The New York Times,* which published a portion of her master's thesis about mixed-race people.

Elizabeth is an inspiring speaker.
On diversity, she rouses ovations by performing her autobiographical poem, "White Chocolate," then invites audiences to explore their perceptions about race and identity. They walk away with a new understanding to never judge a book by its cover.

Elizabeth has spoken at Columbia University, the University of Michigan, GM's World Diversity Day, Gannett, Beaumont Health, 100 Black Men, the NAACP, national conferences, and many other venues.

As a wellness speaker, Elizabeth shares her long struggle with food and fat, and the depression and suicidal ideation that it triggered, and how she triumphed over that with faith and fitness. She talks about how she lost 100 pounds after childbirth (without drugs or surgery) and celebrated her transformation on *The Oprah Winfrey Show*.

Now a certified fitness trainer through ISSA, Elizabeth coaches others on how to achieve a mindset shift as the first step to transforming one's body and life. Learn more on the Wellness page at TheGoddessPowerShow.com.

Deeply spiritual, Elizabeth shares her experiences, perspectives, and tools for high-vibe living in her best-selling memoir, *God's Answer Is Know: Lessons From a Spiritual Life*. She shares how meditation has helped her heal and awaken her most authentic self and serve as a spiritual teacher for others.

As an Intuitive Practitioner certified by Lori Lipten's Sacred Balance Academy in Bloomfield Hills, Michigan, Elizabeth teaches meditation and energy clearing.

In *The Biss Tribe* books, Elizabeth shares the tools that she uses every day to look and feel her best, connect with Spirit, manifest blessings, and achieve a creative flow state in her creative genius zone. This includes a technique that combines meditation with journaling, which inspired Elizabeth and Catherine to create the *PowerJournal*® series of workbooks for self-discovery.

Elizabeth's GoddessMission was born during terrible moments of verbal abuse. Spirit infused her with the peace and power of God energy to cultivate strength to persevere through difficulties, which ultimately resulted in miraculous healing and harmony with her ex-husband.

As America's Book Coach, Elizabeth guides aspiring writers along the sometimes-treacherous terrain of writing, publishing, and promoting a book. Learn more about her "6 Months to Best-Selling Book Success" group coaching program at TwoSistersWriting.com.

About the Author

Elizabeth has taught writing at Wayne State University, Oakland University, Wayne County Community College District, and at national conferences.

As an actress, she plays a major role in the feature-length film, *Anything Is Possible*, nominated for "Best Foreign Film" by the Nollywood and African Film Critics Association. It's now streaming on Amazon Prime and Peacock.

Elizabeth also plays a 1950s journalist in the international shipwreck drama, *The Andrea Doria: Are The Passengers Saved?* The award-winning film is in Italian with English subtitles.

Elizabeth composed an original screenplay, *Redemption*, a gritty drama about a Detroit gangster and a writer.

Elizabeth has been a guest on *Oprah, Montel, NPR, Good Morning America Sunday, The CBS Evening News, Black Entertainment Television (BET), The NBC Nightly News, The Today Show, Tyra* and many national and local TV programs.

Her work has been published in *The New York Times, The San Diego Tribune, Essence, Ebony, HOUR Detroit, BLAC Detroit,* and many publications. Her *Detroit News* articles on race were nominated for the Pulitzer Prize, and she wrote a biography for the Presidential Medal of Freedom tribute for Rosa Parks.

Elizabeth runs, cycles, lifts weights, does yoga, journals, travels, reveres nature, and meditates to cultivate a joyous and peaceful mind, body and spirit.

Elizabeth's life mission to cultivate human harmony through the written and spoken word, and through daily interactions with people, was born when she was one day old and her father baptized her in the hospital room, asking God to make her a "Princess of Peace." As a one-year-old, she helped unite a divided family, opening the door for loving unity for generations.

Welcome to The Biss Tribe

Now through a multimedia platform and The Biss Tribe series of books, Elizabeth continues her mission to help create a better world.

You can contact her at TheGoddessPowerShow.com and at TwoSistersWriting.com.

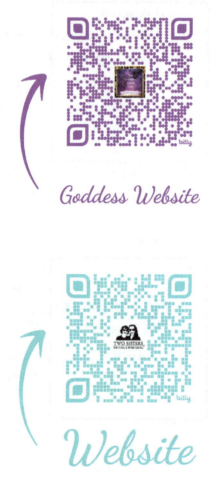

Goddess Website

Website

Please subscribe to the YouTube channels for Two Sisters Writing & Publishing® and The Goddess Power Show with Elizabeth Ann Atkins®.

About the Author

You can also follow Elizabeth on Instagram:
@elizabethannatkins
@thegoddesspowershowpodcast.
And on TikTok:
@thegoddesspowershow.

Endnotes

1. World Health Organization, "Female Genital Mutilation," last modified September 3, 2024, https://www.who.int/news-room/fact-sheets/detail/female-genital-mutilation.

2. Laura H. Smith, "Why Is the Clit So Sensitive? Thanks to Over 10,000 Nerves, First Real Count Finds," *Medical News Today*, October 24, 2022, https://www.medicalnewstoday.com/articles/why-is-the-clit-so-sensitive-thanks-to-over-10000-nerves-first-real-count-finds#:~:text=They%20found%20that%20the%20human,on%20a%20study%20in%20cows.

3. Jessica Choi, "Benefits of Orgasming: How It Can Improve Your Health and Well-being," *Choosing Therapy*, January 17, 2024, https://www.choosingtherapy.com/benefits-of-orgasming/.

4. "Orgasm," *Merriam-Webster*, accessed September 3, 2024, https://www.merriam-webster.com/dictionary/orgasm.

5. "What You Need to Know About the Gender Wage Gap," *U.S. Department of Labor Blog*, March 12, 2024, https://blog.dol.gov/2024/03/12/what-you-need-to-know-about-the-gender-wage-gap#:~:text=Overall%2C%20women%20are%20paid%20less,full%2Dtime%20made%20in%202023.

6. "Frequently Asked Questions," *Kinsey Institute*, accessed September 3, 2024, https://kinseyinstitute.org/research/faq.php.

Printed in the USA
CPSIA information can be obtained
at www.ICGtesting.com
JSHW010711220924
70068JS00012B/1